Hope Over Despair

I0104284

Mariah Forster Olson

H🎗PE OVER DESPAIR

Childhood Cancer and the
Lifelong Journey of Survivorship

Mariah Forster Olson

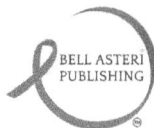

BELL ASTERI
PUBLISHING

Hope Over Despair

Childhood Cancer and the Lifelong Journey of Survivorship

Copyright ©2025 by Mariah Forster Olson

Author: Mariah Forster Olson
Cover Photo by Becky Forster

All rights reserved. No part of this publication may be reproduced, stored in a retrieval system, or transmitted in any form or by any means - for example, electronic, photocopy, recording - without the prior written permission of the publisher. The only exception is a brief quotation in printed reviews.

The opinions expressed by the author are not necessarily those of Bell Asteri Publishing & Enterprises, LLC.

Published by Bell Asteri Publishing & Enterprises, LLC
209 West 2nd Street #177
Fort Worth TX 76102
www.bellasteri.com

Published in the United States of America

ISBN: 978-1-957604-12-1 (hardback)
ISBN: 978-1-957604-13-8 (paperback)
ISBN: 978-1-957604-14-5 (electronic book)

I dedicate this book to my husband, family, friends, and to the childhood cancer community.

And, a special thank you to Cathy and Scott, as well as Bell Asteri Publishing, especially Dana-Sue, Bill, and Lynsey.

Table of Contents

Preface

This story is a deeply personal account of survival, of childhood cancer, and of everything that followed in its wake. At just one year old, I was diagnosed with neuroblastoma, an aggressive cancer that way too many kids are diagnosed with every year. What followed was a brutal journey through chemotherapy, radiation, surgeries, and the harrowing uncertainty that shadows every childhood cancer diagnosis. But surviving the disease was only the beginning. The true cost of survival revealed itself slowly over the decades, in the form of long-term and late effects. Chronic pain, vast medical complications, emotional upheaval, and physical challenges that linger long after the last scan declared me "cancer-free" are my daily reality.

This book was written for fellow survivors of childhood cancer who are navigating lives forever changed by early trauma and toxic treatments. It is also written for parents, family members, friends, and caregivers, those who stand beside us and continue to wonder what it is really like to live with the aftermath. My hope is that this story offers clarity, connection, and a deeper understanding of what survival truly means.

The book is divided into three distinct sections. The first, "Cancer Story," recounts my early years and treatment, how it began, what I remember, what my parents endured, and the moments that shaped my fight. The second, "Medical Issues," details the physical, neurological, and emotional consequences I've faced as a long-term survivor. It lays bare the complex reality of living in a body that still carries the weight of childhood illness. The final section, "Lessons, Principles, and Perspectives," explores the wisdom earned through hardship, the insight, resilience, and meaning I have learned from decades of survivorship.

This is not a story of inspiration for inspiration's sake. It is a story of truth. Sometimes messy and painful, but always hopeful. Perhaps in these pages, you'll find echoes of your own life's moments of despair, and perhaps, like me, you will rise daily and choose *hope over despair*.

Let's begin.

Introduction

It's amazing how quickly life can change from a state of hope, positivity, and optimism to one of absolute despair and agony, leaving us wondering whether a future exists. My parents clearly remember June 6, 1980, as "Forster D-Day," where the "D" signifies Despair, Doom, Disease, Diagnosis, Disaster, Destruction, or any other tragic and negative "D-words."

Imagine a young man and woman who met in high school because they both played the trombone in the band. Charles, affectionately known as Chuck, was a year older than his girlfriend, Becky. Throughout their high school and college years, they were the picturesque example of sweethearts who were deeply in love and certain that they would spend their lives together.

After Becky graduated from vocational school as a secretary and Chuck completed his studies at the University of Wisconsin-Eau Claire to become a teacher, the storybook couple married on June 5, 1976. They secured jobs in the same area and rented a house to ensure they liked the neighborhood and that their jobs were a good fit. It didn't take long for them to fall in love with their new community; after just one year of renting, Chuck and Becky decided to put down roots by purchasing a small home.

They also found great satisfaction in their careers, as both Chuck and Becky dedicated their professional lives to their respective school districts until retirement. Becky served as the secretary to the principal at an elementary school throughout her career. Chuck began as a high school teacher, covering subjects such as psychology, sociology, American history, and government/political science. After many years of teaching, he returned to that same school as a guidance counselor, ultimately rising to the position of principal for many years before retiring from that role.

Three years into their marriage, the couple started a family with the birth of their daughter in 1979. Although she was born jaundiced, she was still a healthy nine-pound bundle of joy who often cried due to colic. The storybook couple embraced their new roles and became happy parents, creating what seemed like a perfect life. They filled their hearts with hope for a bright and fulfilling future for their daughter. However, less than two weeks after celebrating her first birthday, this picture-perfect couple faced a devastating situation. Their thoughts turned to fear, questioning whether their child would survive. In an instant, they transitioned from a life filled with hope and endless possibilities for themselves and their newborn to one of despair, wondering if a future still existed. They are my parents, and the critically ill baby was me, Mariah Forster Olson.

"In all things
it is better to
hope than
to despair."

Johann Wolfgang Von Goethe

Cancer Story

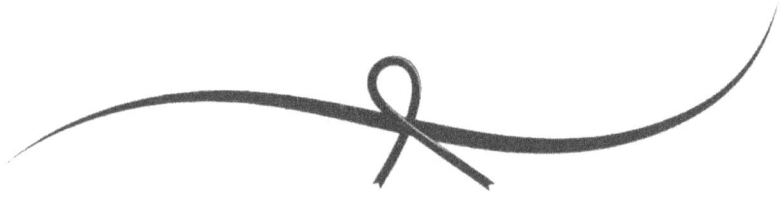

From the time I was born until several weeks before my first birthday on May 24, 1980, everyone thought that I was a fairly healthy baby who simply suffered from colic. Nevertheless, when my mom nursed me, she noticed that I would only sweat and become flushed on one side of my body. She refrained from mentioning it to anyone, except for a few close friends, as she feared the doctor would dismiss her as a nervous first-time mother worrying without cause. To this day, my poor mother feels incredibly guilty that she chose not to mention any of this earlier, but I was her very first child. She did not have the Internet, social media, or other cancer moms to consult with and tell her that this could be the symptom of a thoracic tumor. She was able to explain away my sweating on one side. It made sense because that's the side she nursed me from most of the time. Her body heat against mine would have made me sweat more on that side. I was also born and nursed during the warmest months in Wisconsin. Yes, we have very cold winters, but we can also have incredibly hot and humid summer months. At that time, sweating on one side was not a significant red flag that would indicate cancer.

Information was not easily accessible in those days, and there were no other parents, caregivers, or family members who would have imagined this to be a side effect of a type of childhood cancer called neuroblastoma. Additionally, I did not develop any other symptoms until my tumor grew large enough to interfere with my breathing. This progression is quite typical, even today, for diagnosing neuroblastoma and other childhood cancers. Unfortunately, my case also mirrored another typical progression. It would involve several misdiagnoses before it was identified as neuroblastoma.

About six weeks before my diagnosis, which is referred to as "D-Day" in the preface, I started wheezing and occasionally struggled with labored, raspy breathing. My parents took me to our local medical facility in La Crosse, Wisconsin, where the doctors initially treated me for asthma. After receiving some treatments, my mom thought I had shown slight improvement; however, in retrospect, she was fairly certain that the improvement was just "wishful thinking." My condition did not improve, and during my first birthday party at the Forster family farm, where my dad grew up, I was crawling on the grass while wheezing significantly. My parents took me to the doctor again, and I was treated for bronchiolitis, a lung infection common among infants and young children. After treatment for bronchiolitis, my symptoms improved temporarily, aside from a lingering cough. Then, my wheezing, raspy, labored breathing returned, and my parents and I returned to the clinic. After a re-examination, I was treated for pneumonia, but that diagnosis turned out to be inaccurate as well. My condition did not improve and instead deteriorated with additional respiratory difficulties. On June 4, we returned to our local medical facility, and the doctors handling my case decided to take a chest X-ray.

Throughout my life, I often wondered why it took several visits before doctors conducted a chest X-ray and finally identified my tumor. Had they done so sooner, would my cancer have been less advanced? Would my neuroblastoma treatments have been the same, or would they have been a bit gentler and kinder, resulting in fewer medical conditions during survivorship, most of which I still experience today? After researching and consulting with multiple doctors, I discovered a few reasons why a chest X-ray was not immediately utilized and why these scans are generally avoided in infants. First, bronchiolitis is a common illness in infants and children under the age of two, and X-rays are not necessary for diagnosing and treating it.

My next diagnosis was asthma, but lung X-rays are not the primary diagnostic tool for infants and children. While lung function tests help determine an asthma diagnosis, infants and young children are unable to participate in these tests. Instead, doctors gather targeted, important information from the parents, including family history of asthma or allergies, the child's behavior, breathing symptom patterns during activity and at rest, and potential allergy triggers and food reactions. The physician analyzes this information alongside other factors to determine a diagnosis. In my case, wheezing, raspy, and labored breathing were the main symptoms, and after ruling out the more common bronchiolitis, asthma was the next logical diagnosis. When I continued to decline in health and my breathing problems worsened, I was diagnosed with pneumonia, which was another plausible explanation for my symptoms.

Yet, when my condition worsened, my parents rushed me to our local medical facility, where it was finally determined that I needed a chest X-ray in hopes of obtaining an accurate diagnosis. A common challenge with X-rays for babies and young children is keeping them still, as even a slight movement can make the image blurry and difficult to read. There are, however, some safe, pain-free immobilization techniques that a radiographer can use when X-rays become necessary.

Doctors face significant pressure regarding the decision to use X-rays as a diagnostic tool, influenced by factors such as parental expectations, habits, and the prevailing medical culture. They also must weigh their decision against doing what is necessary to make a proper diagnosis. In my case, doctors followed the general guidelines, which led to my not getting an X-ray for the diagnosis of bronchiolitis, asthma, or pneumonia, as it was suggested that other diagnostic methods be utilized. When we returned for a fourth time, a chest X-ray was deemed necessary to lead to the correct diagnosis.

Upon reviewing the X-ray, doctors observed a "shadow" covering the majority of the right side of my chest. Yet, they did not show my parents the X-ray, nor did they share what they saw or their suspicions regarding a possible diagnosis. Instead, my parents were instructed to immediately take me to either UW Health in Madison, Wisconsin, or to the Mayo Clinic in Rochester, Minnesota. My parents chose Mayo Clinic due to its proximity to our small hometown of Galesville, Wisconsin, and its reputation as THE preeminent medical facility, especially at that time, attracting celebrities, politicians, athletes, royalty, and even "regular" people seeking care from around the world.

Today, the Mayo Clinic operates major campuses in Rochester, Minnesota; Jacksonville, Florida; and both Phoenix and Scottsdale, Arizona. It also has dozens of small clinic locations in several other states, particularly in the Midwest, and they are even located in several other countries. At the time that I was diagnosed in 1980, however, the only Mayo Clinic location was in Rochester, Minnesota, and we were extremely blessed that we lived so close to this very first, original site. Even today, the Mayo Clinic upholds its reputation as a world-renowned medical facility, remaining at the forefront of the treatment and care of its patients.

After my parents decided to go to the Mayo Clinic, they received only a tiny sliver of information about the X-ray results. "The X-rays show some type of shadow behind her lung. We need to send you to the Mayo Clinic as soon as possible. In fact, you should leave today," a local pediatrician informed my parents. They followed the doctor's orders, completely in the dark about what "some type of shadow" meant. They were also unaware of what was coming because no one had shared any other information with them about my condition. My young parents were incredibly scared, completely unaware that this would be just the beginning of a lengthy hospital stay. Thus, they were woefully unprepared for even one overnight stay, and it never occurred to them to return home for a change of clothing or any overnight necessities. The sole focus on both of their minds was to take care of their daughter, and they'd been instructed to get me there immediately. So, they put me into the car and headed to the Mayo Clinic with literally the "shirt on their backs." This all unfolded on June 5, 1980, which happened to be my parents' fourth wedding anniversary.

The doctors at our local clinic provided my parents with a copy of my chest X-ray to take to the Mayo Clinic because, in those days, there were no computers or electronic means available for quickly sharing medical information. My parents vividly recall pulling over on a side street to sneak a look at the X-ray after removing it from the envelope. As they peered through the car's window, illuminated by the sunlight, they could see the outline of a small human torso and the formation of a tiny rib cage. Yet, on the right side of the chest, a significant shadow loomed over that area. While they could observe the shadow on their little girl's chest in the X-ray, they were clueless as to what it represented.

Upon arriving at the Mayo Clinic on June 5, I was admitted to the hospital for further testing. When the testing was completed that day, my parents were informed that I required immediate surgery, which had been scheduled for the next day, June 6. They still were not informed about my possible condition, which filled them with immense fear of the unknown about what could be wrong with their daughter. To add to the fear, there were tornadoes around the hospital and the Rochester, Minnesota area that night. My parents are among the most caring, giving, and selfless people I know, and it was evident that night when they helped move all of the sick children into the halls for safety. They tried to comfort the ones who did not have a parent, guardian, or family member present. And remember, this all took place on the day that I was admitted to the hospital with an unknown medical condition. It also happened to be their fourth wedding anniversary.

On June 6, 1980, I underwent a major thoracic surgery, known as a thoracotomy, to remove the tumor. However, my parents had not been fully informed about my possible condition. In a fast-paced medical facility where you only get a minute or two to talk with the primary doctor or surgeon, it can feel like someone put you into a blender, pressed start, and stripped away all control. Interacting with doctors and medical professionals, it can be incredibly intimidating to ask questions, especially when things are moving fast. Of course, parents gain much more experience talking to medical professionals during treatment for childhood cancer, advocating on behalf of their children, and ensuring their questions get answered.

After I was taken away for surgery, my parents were directed to a small waiting room. Following a brief wait, they received the news that my surgery had concluded. They figured that the surgery had gone well because it was completed so quickly; however, they were led to a dark, private area. There, the pediatric surgeon assigned to my case quietly informed my parents that he could not remove "the mass" in my chest. This surgery was completely unsuccessful because the tumor was far too large and intricately involved to attempt to remove it. Specifically, the surgeon noted that "due to it being a large mass, [it was] intimately involved with major blood vessels and the trachea, making total resection difficult. Therefore, the operation was not possible." Additionally, the tumor grew out of my spine and had grown to extend to my heart, so the cancer was between two very important, vital parts of the body.

Although the surgeon could not remove the tumor at that time, a biopsy was performed, and additional tests were conducted to confirm the diagnosis of neuroblastoma. Furthermore, metal clips were added that outlined the tumor and would be used for radiation treatments to help decrease the size of the tumor, which would make it easier to remove in a future surgery. Those metal clips are forever a part of my body, and if you look at them on X-ray, they resemble staples.

After explaining that the tumor could not be removed, the surgeon revealed that "the mass" was something called neuroblastoma, without further explanation of the term. Furthermore, the surgeon never called it a tumor with my parents, but rather, he always referred to it as a "mass." My parents were unsure exactly what the surgeon was telling them, so my dad asked, "Is neuroblastoma cancer?"

"Yes, and it's a very serious cancer," the surgeon replied. Upon hearing this, my mom promptly fainted. Once she regained consciousness, the medical staff tried to take care of her in the emergency department, but she refused and insisted on returning to me as soon as possible. I must have inherited her strength and fight because five hours after my thoracotomy surgery, while I was attached to many tubes and machines, I was hungry enough to sit in a high chair and eat green beans.

Childhood cancer is the number one disease killer of children, yet many remain unaware of it unless it has personally touched someone in their lives. This was especially the case in 1980 during a time when the Internet did not exist and was not widely available for research; however, it remains a prevalent issue today. Upon a child's cancer diagnosis, parents, caregivers, and even other family members and friends seek to gather as much information as possible. When I was diagnosed in 1980, most people assumed I had leukemia because that was the only type of childhood cancer that they knew existed.

There are more than 16 distinct types of childhood cancer, along with hundreds of different subtypes. Neuroblastoma is one of these, and it consists of a malignant or cancerous solid tumor that affects the nervous system. Each year, approximately 800 children in the United States are diagnosed with neuroblastoma. Overall, neuroblastoma accounts for 7-10% of all childhood cancers, yet it accounts for 15% of childhood cancer deaths. Neuroblastoma is the most common cancer in infants, and it usually occurs in children under the age of five. This is because neuroblastoma can start forming in the earliest types of nerve cells, also called neuroblasts, and can be found in an embryo or fetus. There are even cases in which neuroblastoma has been diagnosed in a fetus during an ultrasound. The majority of infants and children, however, are not diagnosed until their cancer has advanced, when stronger, more toxic treatments may be necessary to save their lives.

Neuroblastoma develops from tissues that form the sympathetic nervous system, which is responsible for controlling various body functions, such as digestion, heart rate, blood pressure, and certain hormone levels. Neuroblasts are present in a fetus, and most of the time, they develop into mature cells. On the other hand, neuroblastoma occurs when these neuroblasts continue to grow, divide, and mutate uncontrollably and end up forming a neuroblastoma tumor.

Neuroblastoma tumors most commonly occur in and around the adrenal glands, which lie on top of each kidney and produce adrenaline for the body. Tumors can also occur in the abdomen, potentially forming a large, firm mass that can compress surrounding organs. Furthermore, neuroblastoma can develop in the neck, chest, back, or pelvis, where tumors can press against important nerves and cause various complications.

After recovering from the news of my neuroblastoma diagnosis, my parents learned that "the mass" invading my body was, in fact, a huge tumor. This tumor grew out of my spine, wrapped around a portion of my heart, and occupied a large part of the right side of my chest. Specifically, it grew from the first thoracic vertebra down to the seventh thoracic vertebra. Just for reference, the first seven vertebrae in your body are the cervical vertebrae, which make up the neck. The next twelve are called the thoracic vertebrae, followed by the final five levels, which are the lumbar vertebrae.

The tumor also wrapped around part of my heart, specifically the aorta, which is the body's largest artery responsible for transporting blood away from the heart to be oxygenated. The aorta descends into the pelvis, but my tumor wrapped around the part of the aorta that connects directly to the heart. This presented significant challenges for treating the tumor as doctors faced not only the complexities associated with my spine and potential paralysis, loss of feeling, and/or weakness in the extremities, but also the complications of the tumor wrapping around part of my heart.

The tumor measured 7 x 4 cm when it was initially discovered, and a CT scan revealed that the mass was also pressing against my trachea, or windpipe (a CT scan gives a more detailed, cross-sectional image of the body). The tumor occupied a significant portion of my chest on the right side and pushed against my right lung, which is why I had difficulty breathing. Since sweating on one side of the body can be a symptom of a thoracic tumor compressing nerves around the spine, I was likely born with neuroblastoma, but it went undetected until the tumor grew large enough to affect my breathing, which happened to be around my first birthday.

I recently requested and received medical records from the Mayo Clinic and the local medical facility that also treated me. I essentially requested any medical records related to my neuroblastoma diagnosis, treatments, and the subsequent medical conditions arising from the tumor and treatments, or late effects. I received the surgical notes from both thoracic surgeries, and here are the details from the first attempt to remove the tumor on June 6. The surgeon reports that an "...exploration of the chest revealed an extremely extensive tumor...It had the gross appearance of neuroblastoma arising from the posterior mediastinum. The lower half of the tumor had broken through the capsule, and there was an irregular lobulated appearance to the tumor. It had grown into the chest wall at the 5th rib and appeared to be growing about the great vessels in the upper mediastinum and impinging on the esophagus and trachea..."

Additional notes were transcribed after the surgery, and after a chest X-ray was conducted. Those notes indicated that the tumor extended from the opening at the top of the thoracic cavity "...to T-7 on the right. No calcification was noted. There was thinning and spreading of the posterior second, third, fourth, and fifth right ribs. Because of the large mass at operation, it was found that the mass was intimately involved with major vessels and the trachea, making total resection extremely difficult." The surgeon then noted that: "After careful initial dissection and evaluation, it appears that it would be extremely hazardous to attempt excision of the tumor, and the tumor appeared unlikely to be resectable since it was growing about the mediastinal vessels and into the chest wall..."

Neuroblastoma and other childhood cancers can pose significant challenges in diagnosis due to their nonspecific symptoms, which often overlap with those of many other illnesses and conditions. Furthermore, children may be diagnosed by their pediatrician, but they are also diagnosed in the emergency room. Due to these factors, along with the fact that symptoms often do not occur immediately, neuroblastoma is frequently diagnosed when the cancer is in advanced stages and has spread to other areas of the body. This typically results in the necessity for even stronger, more toxic treatments because the cancer is far more difficult to treat. The other challenge of diagnosing childhood cancers is that, unlike some adult cancers, regular screenings are not available. For example, yearly mammograms are available to check for breast cancer, and regular colonoscopies are recommended to find or prevent colon cancer, but there are no equivalent screenings for any type of childhood cancer.

Typically, the initial signs of neuroblastoma are vague. They include symptoms such as fatigue, loss of appetite, weight loss, fever, and joint pain. Additionally, I developed high blood pressure and a rapid pulse, likely a result of the fact that I was having difficulty breathing. The other signs and symptoms of neuroblastoma are often dependent on the location of the primary tumor, as well as how advanced the cancer has become. For example, a tumor in the chest can push against the lungs and the trachea, causing breathing problems just like I experienced. If the tumor is in the abdomen, it may make the stomach swollen, cause constipation, and put pressure on vital organs. Further, bone lesions on a child's hips and/or legs may cause a limp and pain when walking. If the tumor has invaded the bone marrow, a child may become very pale and anemic. Finally, a tumor pressing against a child's spinal cord could create the inability to stand, crawl, or walk.

In addition to experiencing difficulty breathing, I also faced Harlequin Syndrome, a condition that may be rare for many, but that can be quite common in children with tumors in the neck or chest cavity. This condition results in the left side of my face turning bright red (Harlequin Flush) and sweating profusely when I get overheated, while the right side (the side my tumor was on) remains completely dry with my usual, pale complexion. On the other hand, Horner's syndrome usually affects one side of the face, and it consists of a drooping eyelid (ptosis), a constricted pupil (miosis), and the eyeball sinking into the eye cavity (enophthalmos). If Horner's Syndrome develops before the age of two, it may result in heterochromia iridis, where the irises of the eyes display different colors due to hypopigmentation, or a lack of color in the affected eye. In my case, my right eye was affected because my tumor was located on the right side of my chest. I have two slightly different eye colors that are quite subtle until you look directly into them. On my left side, my eye is a darker greenish blue color, and on the right side of my body, where the tumor was located, my eye is a brighter, lighter blue. So, the effect is not as dramatic as it could be, but it can startle people when they are unaware and notice it for the first time.

My drooping or hooded eyelid was very prominent when I was treated for cancer, and it has always been a part of my life. It has made taking pictures incredibly difficult because my eye closes most of the time. Each time I had my picture taken, we needed multiple attempts to capture at least one where both eyes were open. The droopiness worsens when I am fatigued, and that just adds to the difficulty of picture-taking. It was also just one of the things that I was "teased" about as a child, but later in this book, this will be examined more closely. As I have gotten older, the hooding and droopiness of my right eye have continued to worsen, and it eventually got to the point where my vision was being affected. Both Horner's and Harlequin Syndromes are common symptoms of having a thoracic tumor, and those effects last a lifetime, long after the tumor has been removed and addressed.

In August 2021, I had surgery to repair the ptosis or drooping of my right eyelid, which is often called upper eyelid surgery. This surgery involves making an incision in the folds of the eyelid and tightening the muscles. The surgery is typically performed on both eyes to help achieve better symmetry. I was not put under anesthesia for this surgery, and it was one of my easier surgeries. The worst part was probably the numbing shots that were injected directly into my eyelids. Directly after my surgery, I was shown my eyes in the mirror, and I almost started crying – I looked really surprised. The medical staff, however, reassured me that this was NOT how my eyes would look in the end, and that was a big relief.

During the recovery period, the main issue was ensuring that I rested my eyes enough during the day. I had thought that I would have difficulty seeing things and that my vision would be blurry for an extended duration. My vision may have been a bit compromised the day after, but since I could see, I overused my eyes a bit during the recovery period. I also had some pretty major swelling and bruising for the first five days or so, and my chronic dry eye worsened after the surgery for a few months. However, after several months, you can see the true results of the surgery, and I was and still am thrilled with the results. I am also shocked every time I look into the mirror and see two eyes that are the same size staring back at me. (Yet, the shock and surprise of looking into the mirror is not reflected in my eyes, like it had been directly after my surgery.) I still have Horner's Syndrome, and the pupils and colors of both eyes still differ, but the ptosis, or hooding, of my right eye has been corrected.

Harlequin syndrome is another rare condition affecting approximately 200,000 people in the United States and can sometimes occur alongside Horner's Syndrome. This is yet another condition that I was born with, which developed as a result of my tumor, and it remains a part of me today. Many people collect items such as baseball cards, Beanie Babies, coins, and stamps, but I, on the other hand, seem to collect rare diseases, which are not the most fun things to collect.

Much like Horner's Syndrome, Harlequin Syndrome is caused by the tumor pressing against nerves in the thoracic cavity, but this is a "condition characterized by asymmetric sweating and flushing on the upper thoracic region of the chest, the neck, and the face," as well as "cluster headaches, tearing of the eyes, nasal discharge, abnormal contraction of the pupils, weakness in neck muscles, and drooping of one side of the upper eyelid." As mentioned earlier, my mom noticed that I would only sweat on one side of my face when she would nurse me, and to this day, I still do not sweat on the right side of my body. For some reason, when people discover this about me, they like to ask if I only use deodorant on the left side of my body, which is the side where I sweat. If you are wondering yourself, I use it on both sides. It looks strange if I become overly heated because I will get the "harlequin sign," especially on my face. This condition causes the left side of my face to turn bright red and sweat profusely, while the right side (the side that my tumor was on) remains completely dry and my usual, pale complexion.

The "harlequin" sign was the most prominent in high school when I played the piccolo in the marching band. Every summer, we performed at a local celebration called "Catfish Days" in Trempealeau, Wisconsin, which lies along the Mississippi River. It would get incredibly hot in the summer and be well over 100 degrees, which may not seem that hot until you are in an unbreathable, polyester band uniform. We would march and play through the entire parade route, and by the end of the parade, all of us were hot, sweaty messes...except me, because I was only a hot, sweaty mess on the left side of my body. This would make me incredibly self-conscious because it was extremely visible and was just another strange thing that I had to explain away.

Additionally, if you were to grab my hands at any time, you would notice that the side that I did not sweat on felt markedly colder than the other side. I believe that is also accurate with my feet, but I typically do not let people grab them. The not-so-fun result of this condition is that I have a difficult time regulating my body temperature, especially in my hands and feet. When I get cold, I get extremely cold, and it can take several hours for me to warm up. This is especially true for my feet, which feel like ice cubes for hours. Then, when I get hot, I get extremely warm and overheat, and it can take me a long time to cool down and feel better.

Typically, once a symptom manifests itself, neuroblastoma can be detected through several methods, and doctors often use a combination of these methods to confirm the diagnosis and to gather as much information as possible about the tumor(s). Some tumors can be palpated or felt upon a physical examination, depending upon their location, but neuroblastoma can also be diagnosed through a combination of blood or urine tests, chest or abdominal X-rays, abdominal ultrasounds, Magnetic Resonance Imaging (MRI) scans, Computed Tomography (CT) scans, MIBG scans, bone scans, PET scans, biopsies of the tumor, and bone marrow aspirations with biopsies.

Doctors commonly utilize urine tests as a method of diagnosis because there are chemicals called catecholamines that can be present in higher amounts in children with neuroblastoma. My catecholamine levels were elevated when I was diagnosed with neuroblastoma, as well as throughout the treatment process. These urine tests are also used to help gauge and monitor the success of treatments, and once neuroblastoma has been successfully treated, the tests are also used to make sure that neuroblastoma has not returned or relapsed.

Checking the catecholamine levels using urine lab tests is very common for neuroblastoma patients and survivors. Currently, some medical facilities will require a 24-hour urine collection to test for catecholamines, while others will perform the test with a one-time urine collection. When I was diagnosed and treated at the Mayo Clinic, they required a 24-hour urine collection. Do you know how difficult it is to collect urine from a one-year-old for 24 hours?. When I would stay in the hospital, they had a special "metabolic crib" that I would stay in for 24 hours, and it was completely open at the bottom, except for a special mesh covering. For this to work properly, I had to be nude and strictly stay inside the crib for 24 hours so that my urine could be collected as it went through the mesh covering and then funneled into a large.

container. My dad remembers keeping me entertained by pushing the crib up and down the hall so that I could see the different sights of the hospital floor, since I was completely captive inside it for 24 hours.

As my treatment continued, we would often have to collect a 24-hour urine sample when we were at home, and my parents had to come up with a way to do this before I was potty-trained. My mom came up with the idea to take the small plastic bowl from my 1980s-era potty chair and put it in my pants to collect my urine. They even came up with a little song that went to the tune of "If You're Happy and You Know It." The lyrics were, "She's got a potty chair in her pants," and they would just repeat it over and over. And if the topic comes up now, many years later, they will become sentimental and still sing it to me. Of course, as I became older, we would collect my urine in a plastic hat that fit under the toilet seat, which made it easy to catch, transfer, and store the urine in a large plastic jug. We would do this directly before each of my oncology check-ups at the Mayo Clinic, and this process has been repeated more times than I can remember.

My family and I became VERY familiar with collecting urine for 24 hours so that doctors could run tests to check my catecholamine levels throughout treatment. At that time, the severity of my tumor and the overall survival rates for neuroblastoma further complicated the success of treating it. As a result, the catecholamine levels in my urine were often tested to help measure and monitor the success of my treatments. These levels remained elevated throughout my two years of treatments, but they never showed that the neuroblastoma was progressing or worsening once treatments began.

If there are high levels of catecholamines in the urine, it does not automatically indicate a neuroblastoma diagnosis. Several different things can affect the test and should be avoided in order to have accurate results. For example, stress and heavy exercise could affect the test, as well as certain foods (e.g. bananas, citrus fruits, chocolate, coffee, tea, cocoa, licorice, and vanilla), certain medications (e.g. acetaminophen, amphetamine, cold and sinus medications, antidepressants, diuretics, insulin, lithium, tetracycline, and vasodilators), and substances such as tobacco, alcohol, and cocaine. Some of these may not necessarily affect younger children, but neuroblastoma can affect older children and adults, and survivors of all ages are often tested. Furthermore, high levels of catecholamines are "elevated in more than 90% of patients with neuroblastoma", but this means that less than 10% of cases do not have elevated levels of catecholamines.

If a medical professional identifies indications of a malignant tumor in a child through a combination of diagnostic tests, it is necessary to treat the cancer as soon as possible. Without any treatment, a malignant tumor will spread, making the cancer more difficult to treat. Once a doctor detects a mass on an imaging study, a biopsy may be done to take a sample of that mass to determine if cancer cells are present. Additionally, a child may undergo a bone marrow aspiration and biopsy, which is where a doctor removes a small sample of the bone marrow and then biopsies it to see if the cancer has invaded the bone, bone marrow, or blood. My dad remembers multiple bone marrow samples being collected from me because he vividly remembers having to hold me still while hearing me scream from the pain of these tests. Some children are sedated to conduct this test, but even though I was only one to three years old, and I did not understand why I had to go through the pain of these tests, I was never sedated for bone marrow testing. The good news about all of this was that the repeated bone marrow tests blessedly showed that there was no evidence of cancer cells in the bone marrow.

Today, the particular genetics and pathology of a neuroblastoma tumor can be determined, which can help formulate the best treatments and outcomes to address this cancer.

In the United States, neuroblastoma is often measured after a surgery, and it is given a staging system from 1-4, with stage 4 being the most advanced stage. There are two other stages of neuroblastoma that are not considered official stages, but they are very important to recognize. Relapsed or recurrent neuroblastoma is used to describe cancer that has returned in patients who have previously been treated for this disease. The cancer can either return to the place where it began or it can occur anywhere throughout the central nervous system. Refractory neuroblastoma continues to grow or spread while undergoing treatments for the original neuroblastoma diagnosis. Refractory neuroblastoma does not respond to initial treatments, and it can be difficult to find treatments that work. Often, relapsed and refractory neuroblastoma may be treated in the same way.

In addition to the different stages, neuroblastoma can also be divided into risk categories to further assist doctors in determining treatments and predicting responses to those treatments. When a child has low-risk neuroblastoma, they may not need immediate treatment, and doctors may use a "wait-and-see" approach. If it is determined that treatment is needed, low-risk neuroblastoma usually calls for surgery, chemotherapy, or a combination of the two treatments. Low-risk neuroblastoma typically has a 95% survival rate. On the other hand, intermediate-risk neuroblastoma typically requires surgery to remove the tumor and cancer cells that are in the lymph nodes. Chemotherapy treatments are given to stop cancer cells from multiplying, and they can be given both before and after surgery. Chemotherapy is usually given over weeks, months, or sometimes years, and the number and strength of the chemotherapy medications are dependent upon the tumor's response to the treatments and the risk category. The survival rate for intermediate-risk neuroblastoma is between 80% and 90%. Finally, high-risk neuroblastoma necessitates using a combination of many different types of treatments, which can include chemotherapy, surgery, high-dose chemotherapy with stem cell transplantation (autologous), radiation, and immunotherapy. Even after treatment, there are medications that children with high-risk neuroblastoma can take to help prevent relapse because neuroblastoma has a high rate of relapse, but more importantly, to increase the survival rate, which is currently estimated at around 50%.

I want to emphasize that there have been significant changes and advancements in treating neuroblastoma since I was treated in 1980. For example, the staging and risk category systems that are used today were developed well after I was diagnosed and had finished treatments. I am often questioned about what stage of neuroblastoma I had, but the staging systems have changed from what they were back then. I also get asked about many other details that are available today, but they were not available when I was diagnosed, and my tumor was never tested for any of them. The only information that we were told at the time that I was diagnosed and treated was that I may have had stage 3 neuroblastoma. Also, looking at the risk category descriptions of today, I was treated according to the high-risk category, yet my tumor was never able to be tested for this because it had not yet existed when I was diagnosed, and throughout my two years of treatment.

After gathering as much information as possible about neuroblastoma and its tumor(s), pediatric oncologists will then develop a treatment plan. Treatment typically depends on the age of the patient, as well as the location of the tumor, the disease stage, and the risk category of their tumor. Since neuroblastoma can be a very complex cancer, strong, individualized treatments are often necessary. The concept of stronger treatments was heightened in the early 1980s when fewer children survived any type of childhood cancer, and the number of treatments was limited. With my tumor being in the chest and affecting several vital organs and structures, specifically the lungs, heart, spine, and trachea, treating my neuroblastoma was especially difficult and risky, and I was likely given extra radiation and extra chemotherapy to treat my tumor.

Surgery is typically used to remove the primary tumor, but often, surgery alone cannot remove all of the neuroblastoma from a child's body, and other treatments are necessary. For example, radiation therapy involves using high levels of radiation to kill cancer cells or stop them from growing. In my case, radiation was first used because, as you may remember, my tumor was too large and intricately involved to remove during the first surgical attempt. The intent was to shrink the tumor through these first radiation treatments so that it could be removed.

Chemotherapy consists of using extremely toxic medications, either injected or taken orally, to kill the cancer cells. Throughout years of treatments, and since I received my chemotherapy regimen, there have been several types of chemotherapy agents that doctors and researchers have found and proven to be effective in treating neuroblastoma, including "platinum compounds (cisplatin, carboplatin), alkylating agents (cyclophosphamide, ifosfamide, melphalan), topoisomerase II inhibitor (etoposide), anthracycline antibiotics (doxorubicin), and vinca alkaloids (vincristine)." We will address my specific chemotherapy medications in greater detail a bit later.

After the unsuccessful surgical attempt to remove the tumor, my medical team discussed and quickly implemented external beam radiation treatments to shrink the tumor so that it could be removed by surgery in the future. It was implemented so quickly that I had the first radiation treatment in the afternoon following that first surgery. The purpose of the radiation would be to make the tumor smaller and easier to resect and remove.

I had eight radiation treatments between the dates of June 6 and June 16 to shrink the tumor, and I received an additional ten radiation treatments after June 16. Each time, the radiation beam was aimed at the tumor in my chest, and the placement of the radiation had to be at the same location. Radiation needs to be aimed at a specific area, and it can be incredibly damaging, so it is extremely important to stay still and not move during treatments. Since this is difficult to explain to a one-year-old child, and it is next to impossible to keep one still for an extended period, I was given ketamine, a strong medication that was used to "paralyze" and "anesthetize" me for each treatment. (For additional reference, Ketamine is also the medication that people call "Special K" or "horse tranquilizers.").

When my parents and I waited in one of the small, private rooms in the radiation department, I found myself acutely aware of my surroundings. My parents remember that for each, or most of the treatments, there was a technician who dressed in a pristine white shirt and white pants who would give me the shot of ketamine. Somehow, whenever the technician would walk to the waiting room to get me and give me my shot of ketamine in the leg, I knew exactly who was coming down the hall and what that meant. I would start whimpering, but as the technician got closer, I would start crying and saying, "No", over and over again. After the ketamine injection, my parents would hold me while I slowly became unable to move. I may or may not have been conscious because, although my eyes were glazed over, my dad vividly remembers seeing them fearfully dart around the room as the injection overtook my body and made me completely unable to move.

It broke his heart to see me become completely paralyzed, except for my eyes moving around the room, while massive amounts of radiation were being sent into the tumor that occupied the right side of my chest. It was also heartbreaking and next to impossible to explain to a one-year-old why she could move her body freely one moment, and not move it at all in the next moment, and for a significant period. Once the injection had a certain amount of time to take over my body, the technicians would come into the room, scoop me out of my parents' loving arms, and bring me back for radiation treatments.

In addition to keeping the patient still during radiation treatments, another crucial element is aiming the radiation beam at a predetermined, precise location for every treatment. This is important because it helps keep the radiation treatments accurate, and it allows for the maximum power and efficiency of each radiation treatment. At the time that I was treated, the doctors helped ensure that this would happen during each radiation treatment by injecting me with a small blue dot of tattoo dye on my chest. Thus, only a few weeks after celebrating my first birthday, I got my first tattoo. We like to joke that the blue dot is a tattoo of the world, and I used to think that I belonged in the Guinness Book of World Records as one of the youngest people to receive a tattoo. To this day, this small blue dot remains my first and only tattoo.

On August 12, 1980, at nearly 15 months old, I had the second surgical attempt to remove the neuroblastoma tumor that occupied the right side of my chest. The surgical notes state that the tumor was "...significantly decreased in size as compared to the previous size mass, but it remained extremely impressive in size and location, measuring approximately 5 to 6 cm in diameter...It had grown into the ribs to separate [them] widely, with some gross erosion being apparent. All the grown tumor that could be visualized was removed...All vessels and important structures were carefully preserved."

The surgeon, however, was unable to see into the spaces between the vertebrae, so it was suspected that there could be some tumor remaining from the first thoracic vertebra, all the way down to the seventh thoracic vertebra, since that is the portion of the spine where the tumor initially developed. A test called a myelography was performed to try and determine this, and the results showed that there was still "viable residual disease" in my spine. In other words, even though the tumor was largely removed, there were remaining portions of it between the spine, and doctors concluded that I needed additional radiation treatments.

The team explained all of the risks, benefits, and goals, and my parents agreed to the radiation regimen. The doctors concluded that the prescribed radiation regimen would consist of six daily treatments, starting on August 28, 1980. In total, I had eight radiation treatments before the tumor was resected, and ten more after the surgery to remove the tumor, which equaled a total of 18 rounds of radiation treatments.

In addition to surgery, radiation, and chemotherapy, there are now additional treatment options available to children with neuroblastoma. For example, immunotherapy uses the patient's own immune system to attack remaining neuroblastoma cancer cells after chemotherapy and/or radiation treatments have been completed. Another treatment option for neuroblastoma is a stem cell transplant. This treatment involves removing the stem cells from the bone marrow and freezing them. The child then receives high-dose rounds of chemotherapy, which kill both the cancer cells and the healthy cells. Then, the stem cells are injected back into the child, where they return to the bone marrow and replace the destroyed stem cells to rebuild the immune system.

There are other possible treatments for neuroblastoma, but many are still in the clinical trial phase. Clinical trials are research studies designed to evaluate new methods for enhancing treatments in groups of individuals with specific diseases. In neuroblastoma, for example, these trials typically investigate new therapies to determine whether they are safer or more effective than existing options. These treatments have not received FDA approval yet, but patients participate in these trials for various reasons. There may not be any other treatment options available, or perhaps the clinical trial is the best treatment option in combination with known, more established treatments.

When I was diagnosed, and even today, neuroblastoma remains a challenging condition to treat. In the early 1980s, survival rates were much lower than they are today, and it was difficult for children to survive any type of childhood cancer. Furthermore, the location and severity of my tumor made it extremely difficult to treat. This all resulted in my parents facing the situation that the current, available treatment options would give me very poor odds of survival. However, in combination with radiation treatments and the second surgery to remove the tumor, my pediatric oncology doctors at the Mayo Clinic determined that I also needed chemotherapy to eliminate the remaining neuroblastoma in my body and give me a fair chance of survival. The chemotherapy that was being used at that time would give me a poor chance at survival, but my main pediatric oncologist at the time, Dr. Burgert, suggested that I become part of a very new "experimental treatment" consisting of a mixture of chemotherapy medications over two years. (At that time, it was not called a clinical trial, but it was referred to as an "experimental treatment," which does not evoke a lot of comfort.) This new chemotherapy could greatly improve my odds of survival and give me much better odds of beating neuroblastoma.

My dad was with me at the Mayo Clinic on the day that Dr. Burgert presented the paperwork that needed to be signed to make this new chemotherapy protocol part of my treatment. This paperwork is incredibly ominous, and it consists of a very long list of all the potential side effects that could occur from the chemotherapy medications. Death was the worst possible side effect, but there were several extremely terrible medical conditions and diseases that I could develop from using this treatment. However, the treatment was necessary and the only way at that time to get all of the cancer out of my body. Chemotherapy medications have to be incredibly toxic to eradicate cancer from a child's body, and each one has the potential to cause many late effects and medical issues both during and after treatment. Furthermore, these chemotherapy medications had, and still have, the potential to cause both known and unknown late effects. Finally, late effects can occur from months to decades after cancer treatments have ended, so the effects of childhood cancer treatments can wreak havoc over an entire lifetime.

Since the original nature of this appointment was just a check-up, my dad took me while my mom went to work, as was their usual protocol during the summer months. My dad needed to speak with my mom before he could sign the paperwork. He called her and gave a very general description of the paperwork that he was given to sign because he thought that the harshness of the possible side effects was just too much for her to handle in detail at that time. I have never known my parents to keep anything from each other - they have a strong marriage, are each other's best friends, and they talk about everything with each other. So, this paperwork was difficult to read and digest, and it said a lot that my dad felt like it was better to gloss over the details of it to protect my mom. After speaking with my mom about a broad overview, my dad signed the papers with a great deal of emotion, trepidation, and worry, and then he put the paperwork in the book that he was reading at that time, where it remained for several years until he finally shared it with my mom.

Many parents of children with cancer face agonizing decisions, knowing chemotherapy can cause serious side effects, even death. Still, my parents, like many others, had to set aside future fears and focus on the present: my odds of surviving neuroblastoma were low, and this experimental treatment offered hope. For the first time, they could imagine me surviving and thriving.

I can't imagine how hard it was for them, high school sweethearts who married and had their first baby just three years later, to sign a form knowing the treatment could cause lasting harm. At just over a year old, I faced likely complications, but without the chemotherapy, I had little chance of surviving. The release form allowed Mayo Clinic to administer the protocol while freeing them from liability if it failed or caused harm. I was treated with four chemotherapy drugs: vincristine (Oncovin), doxorubicin (Adriamycin), dacarbazine (DTIC), and cyclophosphamide (Cytoxan).

My first chemotherapy treatment was given to me at the Mayo Clinic, and my parents determined that it "was not so bad." Everything went fairly well with accessing a vein, inserting the needle, and receiving the chemotherapy. My parents had heard about the horrors of getting chemotherapy and then throwing up multiple times. This did not happen immediately, so they thought that maybe I would be a rare, incredibly blessed patient who did not throw up from chemotherapy. We had just left the Mayo Clinic, and all of us were so hungry and needed some food. We went through the drive-through at Burger King, which was easily accessible on our way out of Rochester. My parents ordered burgers and fries, and my mom vividly remembers how delicious that food smelled once it entered our car. As my parents were opening the wrappers of the burgers, all of our "luck" evaporated, and I proceeded to throw up all over my poor parents and the car. Everyone's appetites were lost at that point, and unfortunately, my parents had to ride back to Galesville with vomit all over them and the car.

There could be several possible reasons, but the Mayo Clinic did not use a port or catheter for my chemotherapy treatments, and there could be several possible reasons for this. Whatever the reason, all of my chemotherapy treatments consisted of as many needle sticks as it took to hit a vein. Additionally, chemotherapy was given to me in one of my hands, wrists, or arms, and I would need separate needle sticks for an IV and a separate one for any type of blood work for laboratory tests. As a very small child who had to be stuck with needles repeatedly over two years of receiving chemotherapy, there were several complications with accessing my veins. First, my veins were small because I was a small child, and I was only one year old when we started, and three years old upon completion of chemotherapy. Additionally, since I only sweat on the left side of my body, my veins on the right side were much smaller because that side had, and still has, a colder temperature. This makes it much more difficult to access the veins on the right side, so first attempts are usually made on the left side. However, the veins on my left side could not be constantly assaulted and needed rest, so it was sometimes necessary to try to access the smaller veins on the right side. Finally, for me and many other people, veins start to "hide" with an increased number of hospitalizations, IVs, chemo treatments, and anything else that requires needles. All of these complications meant that for many of my chemotherapy treatments, I had to be stuck with a needle several times before a vein was accessed. There was one specific time when my pediatrician had to try seven times to get a needle into my veins because they were so small and had undergone such trauma over two years.

The chemotherapy treatments lasted for two years, and they were difficult and numerous. The perks of having cancer treatments at a young age are not having memories of every surgery, every round of chemotherapy over two years, all of the 18 rounds of radiation treatments where I needed to be paralyzed each time so that I would not move, and the multiple spinal taps and other painful procedures. I do not remember the surgeries or the radiation treatments, but I do have some vivid memories of chemotherapy treatments.

The interesting thing about me is that even as a one-year-old child, I was not too bothered by needles, but only if I could watch whatever was going on. At that time and even now, I became perfectly comfortable watching the technicians take my blood or give me my chemotherapy treatments, and I rarely cried, except for one specific time when multiple technicians tried to hold me down during a chemotherapy treatment.

My parents said that I started crying pretty hard and was trying to say something through my tears. Although it was difficult to determine what I was trying to say, my parents finally understood that I was trying to tell the technicians not to hold me down and that I needed to watch what they were doing.

Those particular technicians were used to young children crying and moving around during needle pokes, so their practice was to lay children down and strap them to a table. Then, they could quickly access the children's veins and unstrap them once that was finished. From that point on, my parents would inform technicians that I would be perfectly fine for chemotherapy treatments, as long as I was allowed to watch. As I grew older, phlebotomists, who are the technicians who draw blood for laboratory tests, were always fascinated that a young child would sit and watch them draw the blood. Even now, as an adult, some of them marvel at the fact that I watch the entire process of withdrawing blood, and I do not flinch when they access my vein with a needle.

Typically, giving blood was not a bad experience for me because back in the early 80s, we were given a special treat after each visit to the phlebotomist. We were given a small box, similar to a cardboard jewelry box, that was filled with important treasures for children. These treasures included a sticker, a penny, and a sucker, and whoever came up with this concept was brilliant because I almost enjoyed giving blood so that I could collect my prize. One day, however, they abruptly stopped giving these treasures out after I had been enjoying them for several years. My parents asked why, and they were told that a doctor found one of the suckers attached to his white coat and demanded the program end. It was never as much fun giving blood, and it just became another thing that needed to be done.

I was able to have chemotherapy treatments at both the Mayo Clinic in Rochester as well as at my local medical facility in La Crosse,

Wisconsin, which helped cut down on travel for my parents. Yet, I would have rather received my treatments strictly at the Mayo Clinic because I remember being taken to a large room that was filled to the brim with a variety of stuffed animals that were of excellent quality. For each chemotherapy treatment, I was allowed to go to this "magical" room and choose any stuffed animal that I wanted. I still have a lot of these stuffed animals packed away in totes that consist of my childhood memories and toys. These stuffed animals were such a huge source of comfort and joy during an incredibly difficult, painful time from my childhood, and to this day, I still feel very comforted by stuffed animals. Not only were they comforting to me during chemotherapy treatments, but they were also comforting during other medical tests, procedures, surgeries, treatments, diagnostics, etc. To be honest, they can still be comforting today.

When I had chemotherapy treatments at our local clinic in La Crosse, Wisconsin, my parents and I reminisced about how my chemotherapy medications were transported from Rochester, Minnesota, to La Crosse, Wisconsin. When I had chemotherapy treatments at our local clinic in the early 1980s, the medical professionals at the Mayo Clinic would give my parents the chemotherapy drugs IN A PAPER BAG to take with us and deliver them to our local clinic in La Crosse! I am not entirely sure that they were even told to wear gloves or take special precautions when handling these incredibly toxic medications, and I shudder to imagine what could have happened if there had been a car accident during the transportation of these medications. However, at that time, this was what my parents were told to do, and they simply complied so that I could receive my treatments. How would they have known any different, especially since my doctors were supporting and encouraging this? By the way, those of you who know anything about chemotherapy drugs may need to pick your chins up off the floor because nothing like this would happen today.

Yet, I have heard of this happening in and around the early 1980s with other families at different medical institutions throughout the country. Of course, this would *never* be allowed today.

The worst chemotherapy memories that I have are the feelings of intense nausea. I would get caught between feeling like I needed to throw up and hoping that would take care of the nausea. Yet, throwing up after chemotherapy was such an unpleasant experience because it tasted and felt like chemicals burning through my stomach, esophagus, nose, and mouth. At times, I did feel a little better after throwing up; however, that was pretty short-lived, and I would go back to feeling waves of intense nausea and getting caught between not wanting to throw up, to wanting to throw up so that eventually I would feel a bit better and not so nauseous, exhausted, and sickly.

Each time I would have a chemotherapy treatment, we would arm ourselves with several items in preparation for vomiting. The most important item was a huge, one-gallon ice cream pail that we dubbed the "Puke Pail." I would cling to that large plastic pail and hope that maybe this time, I could skip vomiting after receiving chemotherapy... but that never happened.

My most vivid memory of feeling the consequences of chemotherapy and dealing with the dueling sides of wanting to throw up to feel better, but not wanting to throw up because it was so unpleasant and painful, involves me sitting in a car seat in the back seat of our family car. I was miserable and feeling awful, but sitting next to me, in the middle seat, was my kind and gentle grandma. She was holding and patting my hand as it clutched the ice cream pail tightly. She would tell me that everything would be okay and that I was her "little dolly." I know that my grandma always prayed for me, so I imagine she was sitting there saying some silent prayers as well. She was a very comforting presence, and she and I loved each other fiercely. Unfortunately, my grandma passed away when I was 18, but I have some wonderful memories of her. Even while dementia was stealing parts of her memory, my grandma would still repeatedly tell me that she always prayed for me, for my health, and for my neuroblastoma to never return.

During chemotherapy treatments, sometimes children must take steroids to help kill cancer cells and shrink tumors. Often, taking steroids can make a patient crave salty foods. As a young child, my cravings were always for the same two, very salty foods – CheezBalls and summer sausage. I would eat tons of these two foods, and then promptly throw them up again. It seems silly to keep eating something that would immediately be regurgitated into my "Puke Pail", but this was all part of the nausea and cravings that can come with taking steroids during chemotherapy.

Another consequence of chemotherapy can be losing hair and becoming bald. As a little girl in American society, there is a stereotyped image that you are supposed to wear dresses and have long curls. It is difficult, however, to live up to this standard when chemotherapy crashes onto the scene. As a one-year-old child, my hair had been growing fine, featuring some beautiful light brown curls, and my mother was just starting to be able to style it. However, after the first rounds of chemotherapy treatments, my hair fell out in clumps, and I became completely bald.

Once, while at a fast food restaurant, a rude question was posed to my parents after I had lost all of my hair to chemotherapy. "Is that a little boy or girl? Why would you shave its head?" the person inquired. My mom was extremely distressed and upset, but she carefully responded with, "My daughter has cancer." Luckily, the lady was embarrassed enough to get up and walk away without saying anything else. Another time when we were shopping in downtown Rochester, a saleslady in a shoe store asked, "What is wrong with *it*?" Again, my mom responded, "She has cancer."

During my treatment, an unexpected risk arose when I was exposed to chickenpox. Today, it's well known that chemotherapy severely weakens the immune system, making infections potentially fatal, but my parents weren't warned. Wanting to give me a normal, joyful childhood, they took me to the county fair, where I was likely exposed. When they casually mentioned this to the Mayo Clinic doctors, panic ensued; they even considered flying in medicine from Boston. Ultimately, they didn't, since there was no confirmed contact with an infected child. Shockingly, my parents had never been advised to keep me isolated during treatment.

As the medical professionals continued to severely reprimand and castigate my parents, my mom angrily said, "No one ever told us about this." They were scared and upset enough about the exposure to chickenpox, not to mention the way that the doctors were addressing the situation. However, the next time that my parents returned to the clinic, there were printed signs on the cancer floor warning about the exposure to chickenpox. My mom was a hero and truly made a big difference in Mayo's communication policies. Furthermore, we were blessed because I never got chickenpox from my exposure at the fair while I was undergoing chemotherapy.

Later, chickenpox swept through my 5th-grade class and infected about half of my classmates. The children who had chickenpox were the ones who never had it when they were younger. Yet, I still did not get chickenpox, and to this day, I have never had it. So, I have received the appropriate vaccination and keep it updated, so that I will not get chickenpox as an adult, when the cases can be a little more severe and difficult to handle.

My dad also remembers that there were times when it fell solely on my mom to take me to chemotherapy treatments because he was coaching high school track directly after school. When this scenario occurred, my dad remembers coming home from coaching and holding me outside on our deck or in our living room while I threw up. Yet, the sun would be setting, and, ever the optimist and my first teacher about hope, optimism, and positivity, my dad would enjoy holding me in between vomiting and during the quiet parts. Furthermore, the sunset can produce beautiful images from Mother Nature.

My third birthday arrived on May 24, 1982, but at that age, I was unaware that this was a very special day for another reason. After nearly two *long* years of chemotherapy treatments in both Rochester, Minnesota, and at our local clinic in La Crosse, Wisconsin, my last chemotherapy treatment just happened to be scheduled on my birthday, making it a double celebration. My pediatrician in La Crosse, Dr. Shultz, with his nurse, Patty (who was almost always my nurse too), had been with us from diagnosis to this moment (and far beyond). Whenever I was not going to doctor appointments, undergoing tests, and receiving treatments at the Mayo Clinic, I was seeing Dr. Schultz and Patty in La Crosse for appointments, tests, and treatments. The two of them gave me chemotherapy treatments and helped manage my cancer, but they were also my regular pediatric care team for check-ups and to address any other medical issues. When I arrived that day for my final chemotherapy treatment, Patty and Dr. Schultz had purchased a birthday cake for me. I was so excited and thought it was simply for my birthday, but it was also a celebratory cake for me, my parents, Dr. Shultz, and Patty to mark the end of one of the most difficult times in our lives.

My next hurdle was a *huge* appointment at the Mayo Clinic, where I underwent a barrage of tests to determine the success or failure of the treatments that I received. I cannot imagine how stressful that day must be for parents and their children, knowing that you are either going to hear the best news of your life, or news that rivals some of the worst that you have heard in your life. My dad maintained a detailed journal documenting the tests and his thoughts from that day, likely in part to calm his nerves in between appointments and to create a record of everything, as we hoped it would be a great day that we would want to remember. So, after a long day of testing, waiting, and worrying, my parents had a late afternoon appointment with my primary pediatric oncologist, Dr. Burgert, at Mayo Clinic, who said, "What can I say, everything looks just great. She is one of the few lucky ones. Sometimes it works." He then brought in some of the other doctors and medical students to show them what a "success" looked like because, at that time, there were very few successes and a lot of heartache.

In the childhood cancer community and the cancer community in general, completing cancer treatments and marking the absence of cancer in the body can be complicated and come with some medical terminology that needs further explanation. The term remission or "no evidence of disease," abbreviated NED, can be used synonymously when neuroblastoma can no longer be detected in the body for at least one month. However, remission does not necessarily mean that the cancer has been cured because it could be temporary, and the cancer may return. For solid tumor cancers, such as neuroblastoma, it is rare to use the word "cured" during remission. I was never told that I was in remission or that there was no evidence of disease. Perhaps that terminology was not used in the neuroblastoma community in the early 1980s. Nevertheless, the first five years out from treatment for childhood cancers are extremely important because if these cancers were to recur, they often do so within the first five years from the original diagnosis.

It was confirmed that there was no active neuroblastoma present in my body after my third birthday and my last chemotherapy session. Given the fact that I had been an experimental patient using a new chemotherapy protocol, the doctors were very careful not to pronounce me "cured." It was highly possible that the cancer could return at any point, and there were very few comparable cases since this was a new treatment. During this time, my parents had a lot of anxiety, stress, and worry whenever I had a checkup, and when I had to do blood tests, urine tests, or any other diagnostic tests to check to see if the cancer had returned. Yet, they were careful never to let me feel their stress. After many prayers throughout the five years of remission, my cancer never returned, which was a huge blessing considering the high rate of relapse with neuroblastoma. It was not until I turned eight, which was five years after my last treatment, that doctors finally pronounced me "cured" from neuroblastoma. This also signified a new era - survivorship.

I started treatment for neuroblastoma during the days when medical records were transcribed using a typewriter rather than a computer. Each appointment, lab test, surgery, procedure, and more were typed up on special paper, and then each medical department would use a separate plastic folder to store the information inside. This was also the time when X-rays and other imaging tests were printed out on special X-ray paper so that doctors could put them up on the lightbox to see the images. As you can imagine, throughout being a patient and survivor of neuroblastoma, I amassed a HUGE stack of physical medical records. Doctors would then bring these medical records to my appointments, and sometimes, the stack of records was so large that you could barely see the doctor or resident peeking over the top of them. It also made me wonder if there was perhaps a better system for carrying them into the examination room – perhaps a cart with wheels? There also came a point where doctors gave up on bringing in all of the medical records because there were just too many, so they would just bring in partial medical records or summaries from the different specialties.

The majority of my medical records regarding the diagnosis and treatment of neuroblastoma and my early years of survivorship are physical records, and they have likely been lost or destroyed. Some records have been scanned into my electronic medical record, and while some of these records provide tremendous value, the records are incomplete. Once records were switched to being electronic, complete medical records could be kept in one place again. I think that one of the reasons why I wanted to write this book was to capture and record my cancer and survivorship stories in one place, because my medical records are incomplete and cannot fully capture the medical parts of my story. Furthermore, my medical history is quite complicated, and I have always had bits and pieces of medical issues, dates, treatments, procedures, surgeries, and more floating around in my head. This book allows me to get that information all in one place and tell my story more clearly. Furthermore, I was able to write this book using these memories and my medical records; however, for the first section of the book, I relied heavily on my parents' memories.

In addition, I was also told that the Mayo Clinic keeps and catalogs every tumor, but mine is likely degraded and lost in a warehouse, or it was disposed of because it was removed from my body decades ago. It would be interesting, however, to test my tumor and see what additional details we could glean from it today. This is not practical, however, and even if my tumor were available, it would be massively degraded and well beyond the point of being useful.

HIPAA, or the Health Insurance Portability and Accountability Act, does not have any requirements for how long medical records must be kept on a patient. That decision is left to the states, and this amount can range from 5 to 10 years from a patient's last appointment, procedure, diagnostic test, or even death. This length of time also varies by whether a patient is an adult or a minor and whether the records are held by a private doctor, a hospital, or a medical facility.

Throughout my childhood, adolescence, young adulthood, and even now, I have wanted my case to be followed and studied throughout the years, to help other survivors. For example, I am fairly certain that the experimental chemotherapy protocol that was used on me was first used on even more patients to help determine treatment options for neuroblastoma patients. I also believe that these treatments have been further refined to make them a little less toxic, which would improve a survivor's quality of life. My ultimate hope and prayer, however, was that my case could be used to examine the different late effects and other medical conditions that can occur after treatment, and use that information to help present and future neuroblastoma survivors and their families. I was hoping that my case could serve as an example to prepare others for possible late effects in the future, so that they would know what to expect because someone else went through these medical issues. They would also be able to determine the proper diagnostics and screenings that are needed. Additionally, I would have been willing (and still would be) to serve as a "test subject" and be studied to help past, present, and future neuroblastoma and general childhood cancer survivors.

When a child is diagnosed with cancer, it completely changes the lives of the parents/caregivers and other family members. Often, one parent has to stop working to take care of the child, and this means that the family has to survive with only one income. This makes it difficult to pay the mortgage and other bills, as well as pay for groceries, household supplies, and other items. The other issue is that cancer treatments for children can be incredibly expensive. Even with medical insurance, the majority of families still have to pay a percentage of the bill that insurance does not cover. Chemotherapy medications, diagnostics, surgeries, and hospital stays can be extremely expensive. If your medical bills total $100,000 and your medical insurance pays 80% of your healthcare costs, you would be responsible for 20% of the cost, which equals $20,000. That is a lot of money that most American families just do not have, and this bill is definitely on the very low end of the spectrum for childhood cancer costs. Additionally, when a child is treated away from home, there are additional costs for lodging, food, and gas.

Today, it is wonderful to see nonprofit organizations and other resources that have been created to assist parents/caregivers and families pay their monthly bills or to offer gift cards for gas, lodging, and food when the childhood cancer patient is hospitalized and the family is essentially living at the hospital. Furthermore, fundraisers, benefits, and GoFundMe pages are often created or set up by family or friends to help bring funds in for the affected family.

For my parents in 1980, however, there were very few resources available to help with the costs of my being sick. My parents were 24 and 25, and my mom was a secretary at an elementary school, and my dad was a teacher at a high school, so they did not have any significant savings at this early stage of their marriage and careers. Furthermore, my dad occasionally coached sports to help boost their income, but this required careful balancing since coaching would often take him away from home and limit his ability to assist my mom in caring for me. They did not have much disposable income left after the bills were paid. It did work out nicely that I was diagnosed, had my surgeries, and started treatments during the summer, so there was no school for my dad to teach. My mom has always worked throughout the summers, though, and the year that I was diagnosed was no exception. She was the main secretary for an elementary school, as well as the secretary to the principal, and someone had to be at the building. She also had a little vacation time that was easier for her to use during the summer. It worked out that during the summer months, my dad would spend a lot of time taking care of me so that my mom could work. My dad did not have to teach school during the summer, and sports would not start until closer to the start of the new school year. During the school year, my dad was given a prep period at the end of the day so that he could pick me up from the babysitter, bring me to my mom, and then she could bring me to the local doctor for chemotherapy treatments, and he could return to the school to coach track, football, or basketball.

Additionally, my parents had some amazing friends and family who would check in on them and help out when they could. If I were getting chemotherapy, my parents would always try to bring an extra person who could help care for me. Since one of my parents would be driving, they needed someone to take care of me and help hold the "puke bucket."

During the times that I was hospitalized, my parents were able to stay at Northland House, which provided a "home-away-from-home" for parents of children undergoing hospital treatment. The Northland House eventually became the Ronald McDonald House. The Ronald McDonald House Charities has grown into a massive organization with many hotel-like rooms for families, as well as meals, entertainment, and even transportation for families of ill children. During the 1980s, it was not the massive organization that it is today, but the Northland House was able to provide my parents with a bedroom to stay in so that they did not have to pay for a hotel.

The other organization that my parents received a little help from was the American Cancer Society (ACS). At that time, my parents received a gas card, which was extremely helpful since we needed to travel to the Mayo Clinic and our local medical facility often. They also received a voucher for a free wig, but at that time, the wigs were for adults only, and they did not have any available for children, especially for a one-year-old child.

The ACS has certainly evolved since 1980. Gold Together for

Childhood Cancer, the childhood cancer initiative for ACS, was established in 2018. Every penny that is raised for Gold Together goes toward childhood cancer research, advocacy, and patient support. The money that ACS uses to fund childhood cancer research is in the form of more than 68 multi-year research grants, focusing on multiple types of childhood cancer. I will discuss more about Gold Together later in the book.

We are not aware of who funded the research and testing of the experimental chemotherapy protocol I was given, but it is important to recognize the lifesaving funding and research donated by ACS and other nonprofit organizations. Overall, however, childhood cancers are woefully and tragically underfunded. The federal government gives a small portion of its federal budget to childhood cancer research, but this allotment needs to be divided among all of the different types and subtypes of childhood cancers.

Additionally, many pharmaceutical companies do not fund childhood cancer research. The main reason for this is that childhood cancer is not considered profitable, given the number of adults diagnosed with cancer versus the number of children diagnosed with cancer. This is also the reason why nonprofit organizations, private institutions, and the families and friends of patients, among others, continually need to raise money for childhood cancer research.

The good news is that in recent years, there have been several pieces of childhood cancer legislation that have been passed to help resolve some of this disparity. There are also a few pharmaceutical companies that are focused on developing treatments strictly for childhood cancers. We still have a ways to go, and it is important to recognize that even though the number of children diagnosed with cancer is far less than the number of adults diagnosed with cancer, we need to look at the number of life years saved when a child survives their diagnosis, as well as look at the quality of their lives. These children have their entire lives in front of them, so it is difficult to comprehend, and tragic to think, that profits are often valued over the lives of innocent children with cancer.

I am incredibly blessed to say that I am a childhood cancer survivor, or more specifically, a long-term neuroblastoma survivor. I survived this diagnosis in 1980 when there was a bleak outlook, low survival rate, fewer treatment options, and there was a lot less known about neuroblastoma at that time. Today, there have been significant advances in the analysis of neuroblastoma tumors and what this information can reveal. Yet, even today, neuroblastoma remains a very difficult cancer to treat, and some of the statistics associated with neuroblastoma survival remain quite grim. Taking everything into consideration, I recognize how lucky and blessed I am that I survived.

I first became involved with childhood cancer nonprofits to advocate and bring about awareness and additional funding for all types of childhood cancers. One of my primary goals with my story and this book is to provide hope to families that are fighting neuroblastoma and other childhood cancers because I survived at a time when many children did not live through any type of childhood cancer. When I started my childhood cancer nonprofit work, I learned from families fighting neuroblastoma and other childhood cancers that my story could provide them with hope, and I am grateful, honored, and humbled to be able to provide them with even a sliver of comfort.

As I furthered my work with different nonprofits, however, my involvement became multi-layered, and I was also able to work in childhood cancer survivorship with both survivors and their families. I knew from personal experience that a survivor's childhood cancer story could be just the beginning of a lifelong battle with childhood cancer. So, I also feel like there are times when I walk a fine line between providing the hope of survival from my personal story to patients and families that are currently fighting childhood cancer and revealing the difficulties, struggles, and despair of my personal survivorship story because childhood cancer does not end after treatment. I am never dishonest, but it is important to determine the audience and speak to them appropriately. For example, families are dealing with enough when they are currently facing a childhood cancer diagnosis, and they need to focus on fighting and getting their child through treatment. It would neither be helpful nor fair to frighten or overwhelm others by detailing my late effects from the hazardous, toxic treatments that were employed to eliminate my cancer. Each neuroblastoma case and the tumor's location vary greatly. My situation is particularly unique, as I was diagnosed in the early 1980s and underwent experimental treatments from ages one to three. In fact, one doctor told me that three of the four chemotherapy medications are still used to treat neuroblastoma today, but one of them was deemed too dangerous for children.

As you have read, the first section of this book detailed my cancer story and the diagnosis of neuroblastoma, but the second section of the book will detail the medical conditions and late effects that I have experienced as a result of outdated therapeutics, my "experimental treatments," and the location of my tumor, which illustrates the "despair" part of my story and the book's title. When I filled out my MedicAlert profile, I was shocked to see that I had around 100 different late effects and medical issues that I deal with. In addition, I have had 52 different surgeries, and I have a higher risk of developing nine different types of secondary cancers.

It is also important for me, both personally and professionally, to illustrate the full picture of childhood cancer by delving into survivorship. I feel like I have an even greater sense of duty to inform people about the realities of childhood cancer survivorship and to develop programs to help provide support and information that can assist survivors and their families. I am so grateful to be able to do meaningful survivorship work as the Survivorship Lead for the Coalition Against Childhood Cancer (CAC2). We are creating programs and content that are specific to survivorship and that have the potential to help many childhood cancer survivors and their families, as well as the nonprofit organizations and professionals who work with this community.

Although the middle section of the book deals with some of the despair, difficulties, and challenges that can accompany the life of a childhood cancer survivor, the final section of the book will discuss some of the principles and perspectives that I have learned and that have guided me along the way.

I hope that this book not only helps childhood cancer patients, survivors, and their families but also serves as a source of inspiration and comfort for anyone who has faced hardship or despair and who could benefit from a bit of hope.

Medical Issues

Long-term and Late Effects

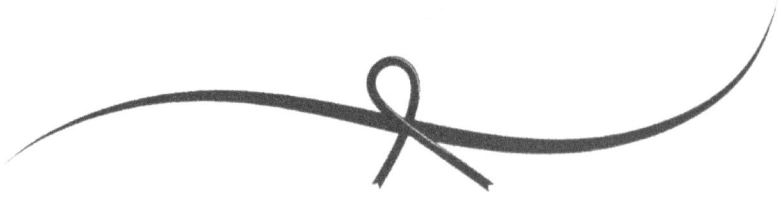

$\mathcal{I}$ was not declared "cancer-free" or "cured" until I reached the age of eight, which was five years after my last treatment. Little did we know that my cancer and the treatments I received were just the beginning of a lifetime of vast medical issues, including around 100 current health conditions, both chronic and acute. By the age of 45, I had experienced 52 surgeries, almost all of which were a direct or indirect result of my cancer and the subsequent treatments. I was forced to learn about elements of the medical field and engage in years of patient education, starting when I was a one-year-old child. I have engaged with a menagerie of medical professionals in various departments and fields of medicine, and have endured multiple screenings and diagnostic testing. I have experienced repeated cancer scares each year, and so much more.

I am so appreciative that I survived, but it is important to note that **_although childhood cancer occurs during childhood, the effects of it can last a lifetime_**. The sad reality is that a survivor's quality of life can be compromised, and the brutal, toxic treatments that are needed to eradicate cancer have the potential to create medical, physical, emotional, mental, financial, and social challenges and difficulties. Therefore, it is important to further discuss the voice of childhood cancer survivors, who have often had to wait their turn and sometimes fight for a voice in this community.

Throughout my experience collaborating with various nonprofit organizations, expanding my network of medical professionals and survivors, and analyzing different medical institutions that focus on neuroblastoma and other pediatric cancers, as well as those with childhood cancer survivorship clinics, I have noticed a significant absence of the childhood cancer survivor's voice. This is particularly true for survivors diagnosed in 1980. At times and in certain situations, I have observed that it can be a long and difficult process to amplify the survivorship voice and ensure that others listen to and understand it. It is exciting to see the transformation that has occurred since I began my nonprofit work in 2016, and I will elaborate on this further. Currently, it is important to recognize that certain places are beginning to recognize and explore survivorship. Additionally, there are other spaces where the voice of the childhood cancer survivor is slowly starting to be heard more; however, it can also be difficult if that voice needs to compete for limited resources with childhood cancer patients. We all recognize that it is extremely important and necessary to treat current patients first. As more children are surviving cancer, there is a growing need to support survivors and address the lifelong challenges that they face. Furthermore, increased research needs to be conducted to find less toxic treatments that would result in fewer late effects and a better quality of life for survivors.

Despite being a childhood cancer survivor with a litany of medical conditions stemming from my cancer and its treatments, the term "late effects" was not introduced to my vocabulary until much later in life. A late effect is essentially a medical issue - be it physical, mental, or social in nature - that arises months to many years after treatment for a disease has ended. Additionally, I also have long-term side effects, which are medical conditions that start during childhood cancer treatments and can remain for months and up to a lifetime for a childhood cancer survivor.

Thankfully, the number of childhood cancer survivors has been steadily increasing. However, it is important to note that survival rates are highly dependent upon many different factors, including the type of childhood cancer. For instance, the overall average five-year survival rate for all childhood cancers is 86%, with the survival rate for acute lymphoblastic leukemia (ALL) at around 90%. In contrast, the survival rate for diffuse intrinsic pontine glioma (DIPG) and diffuse midline glioma (DMG), two types of brain cancer, is alarmingly low at just 2.2%. Although the overall survival rate of childhood cancers has improved and appears quite high, it is important to explore this statistic a bit more. Furthermore, it is important to continue fighting and advocating for money for research to find treatments, especially for those cancers that have very low survival rates, and to develop better, more effective treatments with fewer toxicities and late effects for survivors of all types of childhood cancers.

Currently, our best estimate indicates that there were approximately 500,000 childhood cancer survivors in the United States in 2020, and that number is projected to increase. While childhood cancer survivors are living longer than ever before, our "quality of life" has not improved significantly. That is frequently attributed to the physical and psychosocial late effects that childhood cancer survivors can experience. The number and severity of late effects can vary based on several factors, but "more than 95% of childhood cancer survivors will have a significant, health-related issue by the age of 45. One-third will suffer severe and chronic late effects; another third will suffer moderate to severe health problems; another third will suffer slight to moderate side effects." The National Cancer Institute states that between 60% and more than 90% of childhood cancer survivors will develop one or more chronic health conditions and that 20% to 80% of childhood cancer survivors will experience severe or life-threatening complications from those chronic health conditions, or late effects, during their adult years. Common risks for childhood cancer survivors include: cognitive late effects; breast cancer, especially if there was radiation to the chest; congestive heart failure and other cardiac late effects; infertility; risk of contracting several different types of secondary cancers; joint replacement; hearing loss; and so much more.

As survivors age, they may face an increasing number and severity of health issues. When I was declared cancer-free, we had no way of knowing that my cancer and the treatments that I received were just the beginning of a lifetime of medical issues. Yet, I want to emphasize that although I have many different medical conditions, my experiences are not unique. Ramifications from childhood cancer treatments are horrific. In addition to physical late effects, survivors also deal with anxiety, depression, and other psychosocial late effects.

This section of the book has proven to be one of the most challenging to write because I am peeling the curtain back and exposing my medical struggles and how they affect me. What complicates it is the fact that I have tried to hide the many, many ailments that I face daily and how they affect my life. Again, the reason why I have done this is that most people do not want to hear about others' medical issues because everybody lives with challenges and difficulties, and sometimes it is difficult enough to deal with them on a personal basis. Furthermore, I still strive to maintain a positive, hopeful outlook inspired by my parents' example and Norman Vincent Peale. It is difficult to be optimistic when you are regularly focusing on what is wrong with you. Of course, I have my support system and people I talk to about this because it is important to talk it out. Yet, I try to keep it to a minimum so I have a better chance of remaining upbeat and positive.

Parts of this section flip this philosophy a bit, and that is partially why this section was so challenging to write. I am exploring some heavy, emotional, and very difficult topics. Yet, this is important for many reasons. While our experiences may differ, we can learn from one another and allow those lessons to mold us into kinder, more compassionate human beings. For those of you who are childhood cancer survivors, I am hoping that you can connect and see yourselves in elements of my story so that you know that you are not alone.

Very few people are aware of what my everyday life entails, and I truly have wanted it this way. As you have read before, I have excruciating pain throughout my neck, upper and lower back, and thoracic cancer scar, as well as my sacrum and iliac joint. Furthermore, my pain is in my nerves, bones, and muscles, so it is truly multi-layered. In addition to my back pain, I have many serious conditions that affect my everyday life and take a toll on my body, as well.

Please understand that while my medical conditions are a part of me and they occupy a great portion of my life, they do not define my entire existence. Countless other important aspects contribute to my identity and life. Additionally, to avoid overwhelming others with my medical issues, I typically refrain from discussing them unless I am asked. However, after engaging in conversations with other survivors and working in this community, I realized that it was important to spotlight and discuss some of my late effects to provide another picture of childhood cancer survivorship.

For many years, the medical conditions stemming from my cancer and/or its treatments went unrecognized because I belong to a generation in which many children did not survive childhood cancer. Nonetheless, there were a handful of medical professionals and researchers compiling data and studying survivorship and the many late effects of this population. Strangely, however, I was often informed that my medical conditions were not a result of my cancer and its treatments. which left me feeling like a "freak" every time I developed a new medical condition. Eventually, I discovered that these were known late effects from the treatments that I received.

There were instances when I learned about late effects only as I experienced them, leaving me with no warning or opportunity to prepare. This left me feeling isolated because there was very little known about late effects at the time. Growing up in the '80s and '90s, I experienced profound isolation because there was no internet or social media to connect with other childhood cancer survivors about our shared experiences and late effects. While the internet and social media now offer platforms for childhood cancer survivors to connect, I hope this book will help them feel less alone and different.

Aside from a handful of medical conditions, such as scoliosis stemming from my tumor's location and the radiation treatments, along with possible cardiac problems due to chemotherapy and radiation, it was not until my early twenties that I learned that many of the medical conditions that I had been experiencing were the result of my cancer and the treatments I underwent from 1980-1982. Despite clear evidence from some of the most prominent institutions and resources within our community indicating that certain medical conditions arose from the treatments I received, the Mayo Clinic did not fully recognize that these conditions were the result of my treatments. It is unclear whether this was due to legal considerations or other unknown factors, but that should not be the case because as mentioned in the first section of this book, my dad had signed a document before my chemotherapy experimental treatments that absolved my treatment facility of any future medical issues, long-term side effects, late effects, and anything else that you can imagine.

Without acknowledging that the condition is a late effect, childhood cancer survivors may experience feelings of being lost, isolated, lonely, and frustrated. I can attest that I have felt this way. As a child navigating a variety of medical issues following childhood cancer, I constantly worried there might be something wrong with me, which just enhanced my feelings that I was different from my peers. I acknowledge that for the very early years of my survivorship, the term "late effects" was not commonly used or even recognized, as I belonged to one of the early populations of survivors. Furthermore, these conditions are often referred to as "long-term side effects" because a patient could have started experiencing them throughout treatment before they enter survivorship. However, some of my late effects had already been recognized as known late effects, and it would have been helpful if my doctors had relayed this information to me when they learned it themselves.

Furthermore, if a condition is not recognized as a late effect, we might overlook valuable, necessary information essential for effectively managing the condition. For example, regular screenings may be needed to detect a potential late effect in the earlier and easier-to-treat stages. Without the designation of that condition as a late effect, a childhood cancer survivor may remain uninformed about the recommended screening guidelines, which would detail the type of diagnostic tests needed for screening and how often that screening should be conducted.

I think it is important to address the fact that the Mayo Clinic lacks a childhood cancer survivorship clinic. Although I was familiar with survivorship clinics from my own research and nonprofit work, it was not until my early forties that my medical facility and pediatric oncologist finally suggested that I seek one out. Unfortunately, I have never been to a survivorship clinic, and I wonder how my experience would have been different if I had been able to attend one. Would I have gained a better understanding of my late effects and medical conditions earlier in life? Moreover, survivorship clinics were nonexistent when I was treated, but a select few did exist by the time I was declared "cured" at the age of eight. For instance, in 1983, the Children's Hospital of

Philadelphia (CHOP) established one of the first childhood cancer survivor clinics. Even as I aged and more childhood cancer survivorship clinics were available, no one informed me about them, provided a referral, or even suggested that I attend one until a few short years ago.

Mayo Clinic's pediatric oncology department is tasked with caring for both current patients and survivors, which has resulted in an overwhelming workload for the limited number of medical professionals available. In a pediatric oncology department, the focus should be on the current patients and finding effective and efficient treatments for the various types and subtypes of childhood cancers. However, it is essential to aim for less toxic treatments that limit harsh and harmful late effects. There also needs to be programs for those of us who were patients and have been struggling through life as survivors. Childhood cancer survivors must prioritize their health for the rest of their lives. Survivorship clinics and those who closely monitor survivors help us stay as healthy as possible, while also providing guidance and information about the proper screenings, diagnostics, tests, and other guidelines.

Many survivors, including myself, are unable to access care from childhood cancer survivorship clinics or programs for various reasons. These range from distance, finances, and/or insurance, and lack of knowledge. Yet, having specific documents can be beneficial, whether a survivor takes them to a survivorship clinic or a new medical facility or doctor, especially a primary care physician. A treatment summary is a document that details the cancer treatments that a person received, including the chemotherapy medications and dosages, the location and/or dosage of radiation treatments, surgeries, and any other treatment options. The summary should also list the diagnosis and staging of the cancer and any other relevant information from pathology reports and other testing. A treatment summary can help identify possible late effects, different screening needs for secondary cancers, and other medical issues, and more, all based on the types of treatment that were received and when they were given. It is also an important building block for creating a survivorship care plan, which is a complete record of a patient's treatments, medical concerns, and recommended screenings.

I never received this paperwork during either early or late survivorship. Even if these documents gained in popularity after my treatment and initial years of survivorship, it would have been helpful to receive this information as soon as it became available so that I could use it. It also would have been helpful if the medical professionals at the Mayo Clinic had recommended that I find a survivorship clinic to help me manage all of my medical conditions under the lens of childhood cancer survivorship. Unfortunately, I was unaware of the existence of these clinics until I was much older and working with multiple nonprofit organizations, making it impossible to request something I didn't know about. It wasn't until 2021, at the age of 42, that my pediatric oncologist finally informed me about these clinics, despite the fact that I had researched them when I started collaborating with different nonprofit organizations. So far, I have never had the opportunity to attend a survivorship clinic.

My current medical records are not even sufficient or complete enough to produce a full treatment summary because the chemotherapy records at my treatment facility are incomplete. Those records show that I maintained the same weight throughout the entire two years that I received chemotherapy, which is completely inaccurate. I underwent chemotherapy between the ages of one and three years, so it is impossible that my weight would not have changed at all during that time. I was informed that my weight was needed to accurately estimate the amount of certain chemotherapy medications that I received.

At the age of eight, when I began my journey in survivorship, there was no treatment summary or survivorship care plan available to me, and

I later did not receive these important documents. I simply stumbled upon their importance through my nonprofit work. When I requested both of these items in 2021, I only received a summary of my radiation treatments and an estimate of my chemotherapy treatments via email. That is why I was so happy to discover Passport for Care (PFC) during the summer of 2021, and to work with Ellen Shohet, a former patient navigator for Passport for Care.

The topic of my personal survivorship arose during our conversation, along with my frustration over lacking the documentation that others had. To provide me and any future medical professionals working with me with more information about my treatments and possible late effects, I asked Ellen about Passport for Care and if it went back as far as 1980. I was surprised, shocked, and delighted that it did, so Ellen advised me on the information that I could gather to create my personal PFC profile. I was surprised by the amount of information my family and I had put together that would be beneficial for creating my Passport for Care profile. For example, we could compile a list of medical conditions and late effects that I had already experienced. Additionally, we could list and examine all of the surgeries that I have undergone, and these would also contribute to building a more individualized, personal PFC profile.

My information was successfully entered into PFC, which resulted in a Survivorship Care Plan created for me from the profile. This plan provided me with valuable insights about my survivorship and revealed additional details I had not known before. One of the wonderful features of PFC is that medical professionals can use it to record information as a patient is going through treatment. Once treatments have concluded, pediatric oncologists and/or any other medical professionals using PFC can give the print-out to their patients. PFC also supports individuals like me who may not have received such information in the past and lacked a doctor to input this data into the PFC system. Although this did not exist when I was younger, participating medical facilities can access and input information into PFC at any time. Not only does PFC collaborate with medical facilities and doctors, but it also works with individual survivors who may not otherwise have access to this information. This allows us to provide information for any future doctor appointments, whether it be pediatric oncologists, medical professionals from childhood cancer survivorship clinics, general doctors, or doctors from certain specialties, so that they can learn about childhood cancer and the potential late effects.

I had an appointment with a pediatric radiation oncologist for the first time in my late 30s, and I learned more about my personal cancer story history and survivorship than ever before. My husband and I met with Dr. Mutter at the Mayo Clinic on December 14, 2017. He sat with us for almost two hours and answered every question we had. He also mentioned that I could contact him anytime for inquiries and that I could list him as a reference for my book. It is worth noting that we had never met this man before, but he was wonderful, and he had indicated that he was a bit excited to meet a neuroblastoma survivor who was diagnosed so long ago.

The experimental treatments I underwent for my cancer led to my diagnosis of being cured (no evidence of disease), for which my family, friends, and I are forever grateful. It is an amazing feeling to have played a small role in the development of a cure for my particular type of cancer, and to know that those in the future could benefit from the chemotherapy clinical trial that I underwent. While I am appreciative to have been cured, there is a downside to these experimental treatments and other outdated therapies that I received at that time. Since these treatments were administered early on and to only a limited number of children, the long-term effects of the experimental treatments were unpredictable. During treatment, immediately afterward, and throughout survivorship during my childhood, we were told about a few secondary effects that I could encounter; however, we had no idea that I *could* encounter the sheer number of medical effects that would eventually occur in my body. Most doctors tried to simply explain it away by saying, "Well, it could be from the cancer treatments," but that explanation does nothing to address the late effects.

My most recent pediatric oncologist, whom I would occasionally see and correspond with at the Mayo Clinic, joined the team in 1990, about ten years after I was diagnosed. Since my original pediatric oncologists and surgeons were much older when I was diagnosed, and the nurses and other medical professionals who had assisted in my care retired long ago, this was the last of my original neuroblastoma team to still work at the Mayo Clinic. I thought that she might be on the verge of retiring soon, and when I contacted her in early 2023 with a question about accessing my medical records to help me write portions of this book, I learned that she was in the process of transitioning to retirement. Given the special care I received when I was younger and growing up, especially since there were few survivors from so long ago and because I had been branded as a "miracle" by the medical professionals who worked with me in this department, it is a bit difficult and sad to think that if I would go back to visit, no one would even know who I was anymore.

Despite being so grateful and appreciative that I am alive, my late effects have wreaked havoc on my life. I started experiencing chronic back pain at the age of 14, and by the time I turned 17, I underwent my first of several complex, 10-hour back surgeries. Other late effects had also been diagnosed, and at that time, being too young to remember ALL of my cancer treatments, I perceived these problems to be worse than dealing with the cancer itself. During my adolescent years, I dealt with situations in my unique way, and I tended to think that everything that happened was generally the worst thing in the world. In my early to mid-twenties, I began to gain a clearer perspective and made an effort to shift my viewpoint to truly grasp the reality of my circumstances - the treatments saved my life, and anything that is a result can be dealt with because it is better to have these difficulties than to not be living at all. This section of the book touches on some of my late effects and the medical experiences that I have experienced as a result of my neuroblastoma.

Before I discuss my late effects and medical conditions, there are a few points I would like to highlight. In some of the neuroblastoma nonprofits that I work with, parents and caregivers will often ask me about the late effects that I have from treatments, which always brings about some hesitation on my part. One of the reasons I hesitate to discuss my late effects with parents and caregivers of children who currently have neuroblastoma, or recently finished treatment, is that they are going through so much already, dealing with the diagnosis, treatments, scans, check-ups, and much more. I would never want to add to their worries or make things more difficult for them.

Some parents and caregivers prefer to address issues as they arise, rather than looking too far ahead into the future. On the other hand, the parents and caregivers who typically contact me regarding my late effects like to have as much information and knowledge as they can get. Nonetheless, it can still be overwhelming to hear about my personal neuroblastoma story because I have a lot of medical conditions and late effects. Whenever I am contacted, I try to make sure that the families know that my results are atypical and that I was treated a long time ago. This is to ensure they grasp this context and feel comfortable with my experiences regarding the long-term effects of cancer and its treatments. Furthermore, I like to remind families that I underwent treatment in 1980, and at that time, my only chance for survival was limited to three treatment options - surgery, chemotherapy, and radiation. Today, these treatments have changed dramatically in that they are more accurate, more technologically advanced, and they have been altered to lessen the number and severity of late effects. Some of my current doctors have speculated that I might have received excessive radiation and chemotherapy because, at that time, the primary focus was on saving my life. Additionally, there was no capability to test the genetics of my tumor and determine key factors that could inform doctors about treatment protocols.

Most of the late effects and medical conditions I will cover are relevant today, although there are a few that I may have encountered only to a limited extent or in the past. Furthermore, it is important to remember that my tumor was on the right side of my body, which is why some of my conditions affect that particular side.

It would take a while to discuss all of my late effects, as I have about 100 diseases, disorders, and other medical conditions. As of mid-2025, I have also undergone 52 surgeries, most of which are directly or indirectly related to my cancer. It is a bit difficult for me to talk about some of these conditions because they are quite personal, and I like to try to hide them so that people see ME, as opposed to a bunch of medical problems. I strive to maintain a positive, happy, hopeful attitude, and I would never want to be seen as complaining. While I hesitate to overwhelm you with the extensive list, I think it is important to discuss them and put a spotlight on childhood cancer survivorship challenges. It is important to understand, however, that my late effects are a result of the location of my tumor, the fact that I was treated in the early '80s with a new, experimental treatment protocol, and the medicine and treatments at that time were a lot less technologically advanced. So, I will first discuss the psychosocial late effects that I have and continue to experience. Following that, I will discuss the numerous long-term physical side effects and late effects I experience.

PSYCHOSOCIAL EFFECTS

Depression, Obsessive-Compulsive Disorder, and Anxiety

Most of my late effects are physical, but I have also experienced and continue to experience psychosocial late effects. It is an important distinction to note that childhood cancer survivors not only face physical late effects, but they are also at risk for psychosocial late effects. The term psychosocial is used often in our community, and it looks at both the psychological parts of behavior, such as the mental and emotional aspects, and how the social aspects of behavior affect physical and mental wellness.

At the age of 13, I was evaluated by a psychiatrist who diagnosed me with depression and obsessive-compulsive disorder (OCD). Since then, I have been taking medication to manage these conditions, and I have also engaged in therapy at various times in my life. As I have aged, I have gained insights and strategies to handle my life and mental health better, and I think that my childhood cancer nonprofit work has played a significant role in this process. I find that I can step outside of my own life a bit more and see the bigger picture. While this shift has led to fewer depressive episodes and milder OCD effects, I still experience occasional bouts of depression along with obsessions and compulsions. Additionally, I was diagnosed with anxiety later in life, although I believe that I suffered from it as a child. And now, anxiety plays a larger role in my life than ever before. I think some of this is situational, while some stems from my personality and how I have always been. However, I am not quite sure how to change or alter this.

I think some of my problems stem from growing up too fast as a child. For example, on my first day in Kindergarten, I wanted to take on the role of the teacher and could not understand why this was not possible. My mom likes to say that I was five going on 35. Although my childhood was loving and wonderful, my years of interacting with doctors, nurses, and my parents prompted me to become a responsible, mature child. I was happy and had good friends throughout elementary school (from Kindergarten through sixth grade), and my medical challenges were more manageable because I had fewer of them during this time. Furthermore, I was more open and talkative, and teachers would tell my parents during parent-teacher conferences that I would sometimes talk a little too much

However, everything drastically changed when I reached junior high school, specifically 7th and 8th grades (ages 12-14). At that age, my classmates became highly competitive and materialistic, and I just could not compete. My junior high and high school consisted of students from three different towns. Each town had an elementary school, and then the three towns joined together for the first time in junior high school, which at that time included 7th and 8th grades. Junior high seemed to be all about popularity, and I just was not popular. Once I got to junior high, all of my friends from elementary school dropped me for the "cool" kids from the other two towns. I struggled greatly because I did not seem to fit in anywhere. My former friends all left me, making me incredibly quiet, shy, and introverted. It was so difficult to make new friends because it seemed like everyone had already formed their friend groups, based on past friendships, sports, and other interests, and there did not seem to be room for me anywhere.

During junior high, I sat alone in the lunchroom, which was mortifying. To make matters worse, it became known that I had to sit by myself after an incident when I tried to empty my lunch tray. Someone knocked it out of my hands, causing it to spill all over the floor. A teacher overseeing the lunchroom did not see the other student knock the tray out of my hand, and instead, he yelled at me for being clumsy. He told me that I needed to clean up my mess with a mop that was taller than I was and too heavy for me to handle effectively. The teacher seemed to anticipate that this would happen, chuckling at me in the corner as I tried to wield and manage the broom, along with a crowd of students who gathered to watch me struggle. I tried to explain to the teacher that someone had knocked the tray out of my hands, but it seemed that he either did not believe me or did not care. This was a moment when I felt incredibly isolated, and I had no close friends to turn to for comfort. These types of experiences made me feel even more different from my other classmates. I became increasingly more depressed, as well as less talkative, more introverted, quiet, and shy, which was noticed by my teachers.

Because of my back brace, I could not always participate in every activity in junior high, which made me feel different from my peers. Additionally, I was unable to wear the cool, trendy, name-brand clothes that the popular girls wore because my brace was bulky, and clothes had to be bought to fit over it and disguise the plaster and metal. Honestly, though, you really cannot fully cover or disguise that thing. For some reason, junior high turned into a fashion show of sorts, and you were looked down upon for not wearing certain name-brand clothing. It seems so stupid to me now because focusing on fashion and wearing certain brands is so superficial, and in the grand scheme of things, unimportant. But back then, when all I wanted to do was belong, this seemed like everything. I felt like I did not belong anywhere, in part because of all of my medical issues, and wearing name-brand clothes seemed like such a simple thing that I could do to try and belong. I tried to wear the correct brand names whenever possible, but my back brace just would not permit it.

It also contributed to the most mortifying and embarrassing moments of junior high. Whenever I found myself sitting or lying on the floor, I required assistance to get up, as I could not bend at the waist while wearing my back brace. I felt like a turtle stranded on its back, and it is extremely difficult for a turtle to right itself when it is on its shell. Typically, it requires assistance from an outside source to get going again, and that is exactly how it was for me in that back brace. I guess it was pretty evident to other people because one of my former friends used to throw me into the garbage can during lunch break, right before the bell would ring to signal that class would be starting. At that time, I was very little, under 90 pounds, so it was easy for this girl, who played multiple sports, to pick me up.

Once she threw me in the garbage can, I was like that turtle on its shell, trapped in a sitting position, stuck in that garbage can. I was completely unable to get out of it on my own, and no one would help me because they were scurrying around, getting books from their lockers, and walking to class before the final bell rang. Not only did I have to endure the horror and embarrassment of being stuck in a garbage can, but so many people saw me there because it was in between classes, and of course, everyone laughed at the girl stuck in the garbage can. Eventually, the girl who put me in the garbage can did help me out of it, but on those days, I usually was late for class because she would not help me out until she was ready to go to class, while I still had to go to my locker and get the appropriate books, then race to class on the opposite end of the school.

As mentioned, junior high was an incredibly challenging period for me. Being thrown into the garbage can was utterly humiliating, adding to the ways I felt different from my peers. Additionally, dealing with the back brace was just one more medical problem that I had to deal with. And because my former best friends abandoned me for more popular girls, I was left feeling so shy and scared about making new friends. Eventually, I did, but not until the last part of junior high. Before that, however, everything that was happening felt oppressive, and at times, I just felt like I could not take it anymore.

This was the first time that I seriously considered suicide. I increasingly recognized my differences from my peers, and managing my medical problems became progressively more difficult. This stemmed from untreated depression, along with a lack of understanding about life, as well as the fact that suicide is a permanent solution. At that time, though, believing that suicide was an option almost felt like a security blanket that I could turn to if I ever felt like I could not take it anymore. I had no friends and did not think that anyone from school would mind or miss me anyway. Yet, my home life was wonderful and loving, and my family was the reason why I had never acted on anything.

One day, I became dangerously close to attempting suicide. After being dumped once again in the garbage can, teased about my clothes and the back brace, feeling so incredibly self-conscious about my body and my vast medical problems, and being uncertain I could face one more thing that made me feel like a freak, I went to the knife drawer in my house and picked out a large, sharp knife. I had pictured this in my mind many times before, and I remember just holding the knife in my hand and thinking about what I was going to do with it. I knew that it might hurt a bit, but at that moment, I wrongly believed that the physical pain could not compare to the emotional pain I was facing, which included the pain beginning in my back and other parts of my body. I was trying to think about where I was going to stab myself and in what order. I knew where I wanted to stab myself, but I wanted to figure out the logical order that would work the best, including what would be the most damaging.

I had my hand on the knife, ready to proceed with my plan, but something stopped me. First, I was at home, and I could not leave it to my family to find me in that state because I did not think that they would ever recover or be able to unsee the image of me lying there. Additionally, my dad was the guidance counselor at the high school in my school district, and he had to counsel multiple classes through student suicides. It was awful, and I was acutely aware of its impact on the parents and siblings, along with the student's friends and classmates. I also knew that circumstances would eventually improve. Even if school was not improving, I felt better when I was at home with my family. I also recognized that I would not be in school forever, even though it sometimes felt that way.

For many reasons, I came to realize that I could not attempt suicide, and a big factor was my parents. They went through so much to keep me alive and beat cancer, and they would be devastated if I died in this way. I could never betray them by killing myself, and I always came to them when I had problems. They knew about my difficulties in junior high, as well as all of the medical issues that we faced. So, I decided to talk to both of them about my suicidal thoughts and what had almost happened. My parents helped me realize that suicide would dreadfully hurt my loved ones – especially my family, who loved and supported me emotionally and physically throughout my life, as well as my doctors and the researchers who studied and worked long, difficult hours to develop a cure for my cancer, and who finally had a success story of a miracle child. Additionally, we talked about how junior high was temporary and only two years long, and that I would not be feeling this way forever, or experiencing these difficulties in the future. Also, we discussed that suicide was permanent, and it was something that I could never take back.

Before junior high, I had never sought professional help from a psychologist or psychiatrist. My only experience had been a few mandatory meetings with my school's guidance counselor. In the past, when I faced any problems or concerns, I would talk to both of my parents about them. I pretty much talked to them about anything and everything. Again, my dad worked at the high school in my school district, initially as a government and psychology teacher before transitioning to a guidance counselor. While he held the guidance counselor position during my high school years, he had become the principal by the time my brother reached high school. My mom was also an excellent listener, and we were so close that she could sense when things were off with me. Both of my parents offered good advice, and I was able to talk to them whenever I needed to, unlike a professional, where you had to wait for an appointment. However, my doctors, parents, and I concluded that I required some professional assistance and possibly medication, especially after having suicidal thoughts and formulating a plan to commit suicide.

The professional support I received came in the form of weekly appointments with a child psychiatrist who specialized in helping children cope with cancer and other serious medical diseases. That is also when I was officially diagnosed with both depression and OCD. Depression is a medical illness that causes a person to be sad and generally have a lack of interest in life. Many people experience sadness, but depression involves sadness that has taken place over a long period, and those feelings interfere with a person's day-to-day life. I discussed my suicidal thoughts and the actions that I almost attempted with my psychiatrist, as well as the reasons I was depressed. I also had some thoughts and beliefs that my family may be happier and more fulfilled if I had just died, because their emotional stress and financial burdens would be lessened if they did not have to worry about me. We discussed my suicidal thoughts, and I shared that these thoughts terrified me. I had various images of me doing these acts, and that one time I almost went further with my thoughts when I had my hand on a knife from our kitchen knife drawer.

Because depression is caused by a variety of factors, including genetics, personal experiences, psychological influences, and more, a diverse range of treatments is essential. For instance, relying solely on medication or therapy is insufficient for treatment due to the diverse range of causes. Therefore, a variety of approaches are necessary to address it effectively. My treatment consisted of both therapy and a newer medication at that time called Prozac. However, due to the bad reputation that Prozac acquired in the early 90s, I kept my prescription a secret from everyone but my immediate family. Early testing showed that out of the many people taking Prozac, there was a minuscule number who took the drug incorrectly and committed murderous acts. This was such a dangerous conclusion to draw, though, because that small group of people had also been drinking alcohol and taking recreational drugs. Thus, it was dangerous and inaccurate to solely blame Prozac for those murders.

During the early 90s, there was a huge stigma associated with mental illness, and it was not generally accepted as a medical condition. Some believed that mental illness was "all in your head," and a person should just toughen up, deal with their emotions, overcome life's difficulties, and get on with life. Furthermore, many did not believe that medicine was necessary to treat these disorders. These were such dangerous beliefs because medication and therapy help so many with various mental illnesses. These incorrect thoughts, as well as the fact that I did not want something else to make me different from my classmates, made me keep quiet about my mental illnesses, as well as my medication and therapy sessions. If it was noticed that I was attending more appointments than usual, and I was asked about it, I simply stated that I had a "doctor appointment." This was a secret that I guarded, and forced my family to guard, at all costs.

My depression continued throughout high school, but it never seemed as bad as it was in junior high. In college, it was probably the best it had been, but I think that that was due, in part, to not having my back brace anymore, and finally developing into a young woman. Men were finally interested in me, and that was a huge boost to my self-esteem. I was also a bit more anonymous in college because it was a much bigger population, so most people did not know me or any of my medical background, which was a nice, refreshing change.

Throughout adulthood, I experienced bouts of depression at times that could last from days to weeks. During particularly challenging times, such as when facing a serious medical problem, these periods could extend to several months. As I have become older, I have been able to put my life into perspective a bit more, and that has helped lessen the number and severity of my episodes of depression. Furthermore, I strive to focus on hope, optimism, and positivity. Sometimes this can help me through my depressive state, but sometimes my mental health just does not allow me to focus on this. I know it is important for a person to feel the full spectrum of emotions throughout life. If you do not know what devastation and sadness feel like, how will you be able to process and know how wonderful joy, happiness, and delight feel?

While it is essential to experience this range of emotions, if I become depressed, I need to address it and try to work through it fairly quickly because the longer that I am in that state, the more difficult it is to come out of it. This is detrimental not only for me but, more importantly, for my loved ones if I remain in a prolonged state of depression. As I grew older, it became somewhat easier to manage my emotions appropriately thanks to the real-life experiences I could draw upon and utilize. It is also important to remember to keep life and emotions in perspective and not jump around from one extreme emotion to the next. All of this typically gets easier and more manageable with age, but it is so important to seek out mental health help if things do not feel easier and depression gets out of control.

Since junior high and high school, I have contemplated suicide, especially when my chronic pain is severe. It has been difficult to navigate life with this many medical conditions. However, I have never been as close to attempting suicide as I was when I was in junior high with my hand on a sharp knife. I have concocted some half-hearted plans about how I could commit suicide, but I never forgot the reasons why I could not follow through with those plans. I could not do that to my family, and I still wholeheartedly believe that "Suicide is a permanent solution to a temporary problem."

In addition to depression, I was diagnosed with OCD. This disorder is characterized by frequent thoughts called obsessions. To cope with these upsetting, intrusive, repetitive thoughts, a person feels an urge to repeat certain rituals or behaviors, called compulsions. Many people, for example, might take a moment to double-check that the door is locked or the curling iron is turned off. In contrast, a person with OCD could be bombarded with thoughts about checking to see that the door is locked, and then they may repeatedly lock and unlock the door over and over again to alleviate these thoughts. Obsessive-compulsive disorder is only considered when these thoughts and rituals disrupt an individual's daily life. This medical illness must be diagnosed by a doctor. A widely known example of OCD includes washing hands repeatedly, and possibly even washing them so much that they become dry, cracked, and start bleeding, yet the obsession and compulsion continue.

My OCD caused me to do things in a certain way and order, and at a certain time, and if anyone disrupted this schedule, I would become very upset, and extremely agitated, often striving to return to the original schedule I had set for myself. I also had a problem with rumination – thinking the same thoughts over and over again. For example, I took music lessons throughout elementary, junior high, and high school, and it is essential to practice daily to progress and enhance your skills.

Throughout most of my education, I took piano lessons and oboe lessons. I made it a point to practice immediately, ensuring it was incorporated into the day. This way, the rest of the day would be open for studying or doing something fun. Even if I had the whole day in front of me with nothing else planned, I had to practice my instruments right away. Sometimes, though, my parents had chores or other things for me to do before I could practice. This felt like the worst thing in the world because I had planned to practice first, so I needed to follow through with that and finish it before I could move on to the next task. Of course, I had plenty of time to complete everything I wanted to in the day. Even on busy days, when I had much more than just practicing to do, I would worry about getting everything finished, but my mom would repeatedly say, "You always finish everything that you want to in the day, so calm down." However, my compulsions and obsessions about my schedule and practicing controlled my life, and I got very upset with my parents if they did not let me stick to my schedule.

As a child, I was also very meticulous about maintaining cleanliness and orderliness in my bedroom and with my toys. My bedroom represented my personal space as a child, and it was where I could control what everything looked like. I was "that child" who would instantly pick up and throw away a clean tissue if it fell on the floor of my bedroom, as I believed it would turn my entire room into "a mess." For many years, my Barbies lived in my bedroom with me in a large Barbie house that my mom had lovingly made for me. Constructed from wood, the house featured carpet and wallpaper, along with paint and tiny pictures that adorned the walls. As you can imagine, my Barbie house and all of the accessories were kept in immaculate condition. I played with my Barbies, but I rarely, if ever, lost any of the tiny accessories.

When I was in elementary school, I hosted a sleepover with two of my friends. We all slept in my room, and the next morning I awoke to find them both playing Barbies. Not quite ready to rise, I lay there listening to my friends playing. There was not much going on, but it seemed that my friends were expecting me to wake up soon because they started putting the Barbies away. I remember hearing one of them say, "Make sure you put everything back exactly how we got it because Mariah will FREAK OUT if it looks different." On one hand, I appreciated that they would do that for me, but on the other hand, I was a bit embarrassed. Shortly after they put everything back in what they thought was the same position, I decided to "wake up." My friends told me that they had played with my Barbies, but they put everything back how I had originally had it. I attempted to ignore the differences in the Barbie house and played it off really cool and said, "No problem." Then, I tried to wait until they left before moving everything back to its original location, although I am not sure if I was successful at waiting.

When I was in college, the OCD only extended to my side of the dorm room or my bedroom in a shared apartment. However, once my husband and I got our own apartment together, I had to learn to be okay with a little mess. My husband did NOT grow up keeping his bedroom clean and tidy, but he sure tried to adjust and become better about keeping things clean when he dated me so that I would feel more comfortable. When we first lived together and for the first years of our marriage, I was a bit more able-bodied than I am today. This meant that I would make the time to clean our small apartment EVERY OTHER DAY, which I know is very excessive. However, my OCD made me feel unsettled and like the house was a messy disaster on the days that I did not clean it.

I have always had a cat, and my husband got a package deal when he married me – my cat, Dolce, and I needed to stay together. Indoor cats always come with a litter box, and when I lived at home with my parents, the litter box was in the basement in a storage room. Apartment living, however, does not come with a basement, so we had to put the litter box in a closet. Every inch of a small apartment matters, so litter on the floor became an everyday occurrence. Dolce had a beautiful, long fur coat, so sometimes the litter would get stuck in her fur when she was in the litter box. Plus, it is just natural that the small, clumpable litter escapes the litter box. However, my OCD became so bad at one point that I would cry when I found litter outside of the litter box because, in my mind, it made the entire house messy. Today, we use the *Breeze Litter Box System*, which consists of pads that catch the urine and large pellets in place of small, clumpable litter. Now, we only occasionally find a litter pellet outside of the litter box, and they are so easy to clean up.

I was a huge perfectionist, and I needed to do things a certain way to a certain degree of neatness and precision. This carried over into my schoolwork, and it continued with me throughout my secondary, undergraduate, and graduate schooling. It was worse, however, in junior high and high school because I was determined to be the valedictorian of my graduating class. We had several highly intelligent people in my class, and people assumed that they would be at the top of our class. I, on the other hand, was also a good student, but I did not mention that at school. When it was announced that I was the valedictorian for the class of 1997 at Galesville-Ettrick-Trempealeau High School, people were surprised because it was a bit unexpected. The goal of becoming valedictorian forced me to study fiercely and spend lots of time on my schoolwork. When my perfect "A" average was marred by an "A-" in Geometry, I was so upset and cried for days because I thought that I had lost the valedictorian title for good. Luckily, that was not the case, and I achieved my goal, graduating as our high school class valedictorian.

It was not until my thirties that I was diagnosed with anxiety, though I highly suspect that I have had anxiety my entire life. I was a very anxious child, and I worried about everything. It was difficult for me to try new things without thinking through them, going through all the scenarios, and worrying about the outcome. The anxiety started at an early age, but one of the earliest forms of serious anxiety that I remember was when I was in elementary school, and I had to travel to Chicago to see a new doctor who could potentially help me with my sinus problems and headaches. I had never been to Chicago before, but being from Galesville, Wisconsin, an incredibly small town of around 1,300 people, I was nervous to go to such a big place. All I knew about Chicago came from television, where I had seen a significant amount of crime and murders in the city and its surrounding suburbs. That was all that I could think about, and I could not sleep the night before my dad and I left for Chicago. Each time we had to travel to Chicago, I was convinced that someone would try to murder my dad and me. I was in tears, butterflies filled my stomach, and I could not think about anything else. However, the idea that perhaps my headaches and sinus pain could be helped by traveling there forced me into taking these trips. All I wanted was some relief, but that was not enough to stop the anxieties and the worries about Chicago.

My anxiety stayed pretty high throughout elementary, junior high, and high school, but it was a bit more manageable throughout college and my twenties. I met my husband, Troy, a few months before I turned 22. He was, and still is, very relaxed, carefree, with a "go-with-the-flow" attitude. Throughout our relationship, we rubbed off on each other a bit, and I became just a tiny bit more relaxed and carefree. My OCD became less severe, and I think that Troy, my medication, and my life experiences helped me with this. Even my family has noticed that today, I am somewhat more relaxed about certain things, and some of my obsessions and compulsions have improved. That is not to say that OCD has disappeared because it has reared its ugly head throughout my life; however, it is not necessarily the most prominent and pressing issue. That spot is reserved for anxiety, which has just heightened and worsened throughout my thirties and beyond to the present day.

At times, I find myself overwhelmed with worry, nervousness, and restlessness, and I have trouble relaxing or sleeping. I try to stay busy most of the time so that I can focus my energies on other things. Yet, it can be quite exhausting to try and fill up my hours with work and activities because I require rest due to my medical concerns. My mind and body know this, but the worry and anxiety take over and push everything else out of my mind.

I am also incredibly self-conscious when I am out in public, and I frequently worry about what other people think of me, both physically and mentally. I have to carefully do my makeup and hair, and select an outfit that I feel comfortable and good in, not because I am vain, but because I cut down on these worries a tiny bit if I feel like I look my best. I often feel like I am "acting" or "putting on a show" when I am out in public because I try to be very careful with what I say in front of people about my medical problems. Once I feel comfortable with someone, that melts away, allowing me to be more comfortable, open, and authentic. Yet, until that time comes, it can be quite exhausting to play and be the best version of myself when I am typically nervous and anxious, as well as exhausted and dealing with a menagerie of medical troubles.

Having anxiety and depression, as well as OCD, I feel like my life can sometimes be one of contradictions. Anxiety makes me feel like a clock or music box, wound up almost as tight as can be, full of worries and never having a moment of reprieve. Honestly, I feel like I am worrying all the time, and that worry started sometime when I was a child. The only day as an adult that I remember when I had no worries was when I had to take Klonopin or Xanax® for a medical test. It made me a little drowsy/loopy, but it also took those worries away. It was wonderful and I felt so happy and carefree. It was like I was living in a completely different world. Remember how the *Wizard of Oz* switched from black-and-white to color? That is sort of how it felt to me when my worries and anxieties were obliterated by the Xanax®. However, I did not want to be on something that altered my mood so much and that could be habit-forming. My doctor agreed that he did not want to prescribe Xanax® because it could be addictive. I am currently on an anti-anxiety medication that is not as effective, but it is also not addictive and is safer to use.

Anxiety also makes me worry about what others think of me. All. The. Time. Depression and dealing with my medical issues, on the other hand, can make me exhausted, and at times, it will limit what I can do. Then, my anxiety resurfaces, reminding me of looming deadlines and the responsibilities that others rely on me for, whether it's work commitments or various social events. This creates an ongoing struggle between these conflicting emotions. I also worry about people finding out about my OCD because there is so much stigma around it, and my particular case does not follow what people commonly think of when they ponder this mental health concern. Yet, it does affect me and can sometimes slow things down because I need to work on it in a slow, deliberate way.

Really, though, the anxiety and depression battle each other in my mind quite a bit. When I cannot attend a social gathering with my husband, there is usually a particular reason for it. However, I feel incredibly guilty staying home, and I worry about what he thinks, as well as what others think when I am unable to be there. Sure, it is good to be home because I do not have to put on an act and pretend like I feel fantastic, or I can get a little work done and feel productive about myself. The process of getting ready to go somewhere and then going to that place can be so exhausting. And to be honest, I would probably get a lot more out of staying at home and resting with my cat, Isaac, who is always happy to be with me and lets me watch whatever I want to on television. (More about Isaac, my Siamese cat, in the next section.) Plus, I always have so much work to concentrate on, and going out for even a little bit sets me back the next day. Given the extensive workload I have, I require as much time as possible to focus on my tasks. I feel better being at home and resting because I would have been horrible company anyway. And, this just brings me back again to disappointing people because I had to miss a get-together. Plus, I know that it is good to get out of the house and do something that is not work. AAAAAHHHHH. I wish that I could shut off those voices in my head, but my OCD and ruminations are way too active for this to happen most of the time. And, my anxiety and depression like playing off of each other too much to silence things right at the source.

As you have read, one of my primary perspectives is to approach life with a positive, optimistic attitude. However, like everyone else, I feel a wide range of emotions. I have battled depression and OCD, along with anxiety, so I also have experienced the emotions that come with these conditions. I think that it is crucial to recognize that mental health issues exist in our community, from patients and survivors to parents, caregivers, siblings, other family members, and even medical professionals. Additionally, it is important to understand that maintaining hope, optimism, and positivity at all times is not realistic. Everyone experiences days when they feel down, or they experience the pain and difficulties that accompany life, whether that pain is physical, mental, or emotional, and this can affect how happy one may feel on any given day.

The important part is that after experiencing a period of feeling down, your next response is critical. While someone can't maintain a positive, happy, optimistic outlook all the time, my message is to strive for this perspective on life. If I stay in a sad, depressed state for too long, it becomes more difficult to overcome these feelings and this mentality. It is always important to let yourself feel the full spectrum of emotions, but once you allow yourself to feel angry, sad, or down, it is so important to shift towards feeling better and happier while focusing on the positive aspects of life. No matter the situation, I am convinced that there is something hopeful or positive that you can learn or realize, no matter how small that may be.

PHYSICAL SIDE EFFECTS & LATE EFFECTS

In addition to the psychosocial late effects that childhood cancer survivors may experience, there is an array of physical side effects and late effects they may also encounter. In this next section, I will detail some of the physical side effects and late effects I have personally faced, many of which I will continue to experience for the rest of my life. I cannot possibly detail every medical condition that I have encountered, but I will do my best to give an overall view of my medical conditions. Some of them are common among childhood cancer survivors, but others are quite strange and unique to me, my tumor and its location, or to neuroblastoma.

Horner's Syndrome

Since my tumor was on the right side, my right eye has Horner's Syndrome, which, as mentioned previously, means that the pupil and overall size of one of my eyes is smaller than the other. For me, this results in a constricted pupil and drooping on the right side, which is even more pronounced when I am tired. Many people with thoracic tumors can develop Horner's Syndrome because the nerves controlling this area are located in the thoracic cavity.

My drooping eyelid was very prominent when I was treated for cancer, and it had always been a part of my life. It has made taking pictures incredibly difficult because my right eye closes most of the time, especially when there is a flash. Capturing a picture where both eyes are open often requires multiple attempts. The droopiness worsens when I am fatigued, which just adds to the difficulty of picture-taking. And my family loves taking pictures. It was also a source of teasing when I was a child. As I have grown older, the hooding and droopiness of my eye have progressively worsened, ultimately affecting my vision.

In August 2021, I underwent surgery to repair the ptosis or drooping of my right eyelid, commonly referred to as upper eyelid surgery. This surgery involves making an incision along the folds of the eyelid and tightening the muscles. Instead of just performing the surgery on the affected eye, it is performed on both eyes to help achieve better symmetry. I was not put under anesthesia for this surgery, and it was one of my easier surgeries. The worst part was probably the numbing shots that were injected directly into my eyelids. Directly after my surgery, I was shown my eyes in the mirror, and I almost started crying – I looked really surprised, similar to celebrities who had bad plastic surgery. The medical staff, however, assured me that this was NOT how my eyes would look in the end, and that was a HUGE relief.

During the recovery period, the main issue was ensuring that I rested my eyes enough during the day. I had thought that I would struggle with my eyesight and that my vision would be blurry for an extended period. My vision may have been a bit compromised the day after, but since I could see, I overused my eyes a bit during the initial recovery period. I also had some pretty major swelling and bruising for the first five days or so, and my chronic dry eye worsened after the surgery. However, after several months, I could see the true results of the surgery, and I was thrilled. I am also surprised every time I look into the mirror and see two eyes that are the same size staring back at me (Yet, the shock and surprise of looking into the mirror is not reflected in my eyes, like it had been directly after my surgery.) I still have Horner's Syndrome, and the pupils and colors of both of my eyes still differ, but the ptosis of my right eye has been corrected, and it now matches my left eye. So, now, when I ruin pictures, it is because BOTH eyes are shut, rather than just my right eye.

Harlequin Syndrome and Asymmetric Flushing

Harlequin Syndrome and asymmetric flushing are common symptoms associated with the diagnosis of neuroblastoma tumors located in the thoracic region. This occurs because the affected nerves come down into the chest and are influenced by the tumor. At birth, I began sweating on one side of my body, but no one told my parents that this could be a symptom of childhood cancer. Today, despite the removal of my tumor, I still experience harlequin syndrome and asymmetric flushing because the nerves were irreparably affected. I only sweat and flush on one side of my body, so it can be difficult for my body to regulate and get accustomed to extreme hot and cold weather. Essentially, I have two different climate zones on my body, with my right side always being colder than my left side because that is the side that I do not sweat on. As previously mentioned, the "harlequin" sign was the most prominent in those high school marching band days when I became a hot, sweaty mess only on my left side, causing me to feel very self-conscious.

If you were to grab my hands at almost any moment, you'd notice a stark difference. One side would feel significantly colder than the other due to my lack of sweating on that side. I suspect the same is true for my feet, though I don't usually let people test that theory. One of the more frustrating effects of this condition is how poorly I regulate my body temperature, especially in my hands and feet. When I get cold, I get cold, and it can take hours to warm back up—my feet often feel like ice cubes for what seems like forever. On the flip side, when I overheat, I get really hot, and it takes just as long to cool down and feel normal again. One time, I got a pedicure and they were advertising this new nail polish that was two different colors – it was one color when your body was warm or the sun was shining on it, and another color when your body was cooler or in colder temperatures. At least, that is how it was supposed to work. My nail polish was always two different colors because my right side was cooler and did not sweat, but the other side was warmer and would be another color. I decided that I would never get this type of nail polish again because I have always been a person who **NEEDS** to match, and having two different colors of nail polish on my toes was a little too much for me to handle. Just like Horner's Syndrome, I still have Harlequin Syndrome and asymmetric flushing, and I will have both for the rest of my life.

Growing up, I felt very alone because I had never met another child who had cancer, much less the same type of cancer I had, with the same long-term side effects and late effects. I had met plenty of adults who had cancer, but never a child. Before the internet came into existence, I had no way to connect with other survivors like this, and my local hospital also lacked a survivorship clinic. So, to help me feel more accepted and connected to the childhood cancer community, my parents purchased a book for me titled "I Want to Grow Hair, I Want to Grow Up, I Want to Go to Boise," by Erma Bombeck, an American humorist and bestselling author. The book is about children fighting cancer with humor and hope. In the book, there was a story about a boy named Ryan who had neuroblastoma in the thoracic area, just like I had. The book also had a picture that Ryan drew, depicting himself as a frog with a thoracic scar. This frog was colored in with two different shades of green, and it was talking to a second frog, which was only one shade of green and meant to represent a healthy frog. The two-toned frog was meant to illustrate and show that Ryan had Harlequin Syndrome and asymmetric sweating and flushing on one side of the body. The two-toned frog explained to the healthy frog, "There is nothing wrong with me. I just had cancer." When I first read this book, I had never met or even known about another neuroblastoma survivor. Neither my local medical clinic nor the facility where I was treated had a survivorship clinic. It was wonderful and pretty life-changing for me to read about someone who had neuroblastoma in the thoracic area, as well as someone who experienced some of the strange long-term side effects like I did. Finally, it was confirmed that there was someone out there like me!

Cardiac Issues

I was made aware of the possible cardiac issues that I could experience due to the chemotherapy I received. I had a type of chemotherapy medication called an anthracycline, which can cause children to have cardiac problems immediately or later in life. Specifically, I was given doxorubicin, which is a type of anthracycline that is used to treat many different types of cancers; however, this class of medication has been shown to cause cardiac problems. That medication was administered in the early 80s, and part of my ongoing monitoring from that treatment is to regularly undergo an echocardiogram and an EKG (electrocardiogram), as well as regular appointments with a cardiologist, to make sure that my heart was functioning properly.

When we consulted with Dr. Mutter, he let us know that the carotid artery was in the radiation field, so the general radiation that I had to my chest area also increased the risk of cardiac late effects. It was not until much later, after talking to Dr. Mutter, that I realized the potential seriousness of the issues arising from the radiation treatments. Direct radiation to the chest can also give children cardiac problems, and we were never informed about this risk. Overall, I like to say that I got a double whammy dose of both chemotherapy and radiation to the chest, so you would think that I would undoubtedly have heart issues, right? Believe it or not, I do not have any cardiac issues at this time. It is a bit surprising because this can be a common late effect for childhood cancer survivors who are treated similarly to me. There is always the potential to have cardiac issues in the future, so I need to continue to be regularly monitored and tested.

In September 2021, I participated as a panelist in the Externally-Led Patient Focused Drug Development (EL-PFDD) meeting on childhood cancer and cardiac toxicity, hosted by Children's Cancer Cause. The purpose of these types of meetings is to provide the Food and Drug Administration (FDA) with the patient's perspective about specific diseases and their treatments. This is one of the only chances for the FDA to hear the voice of the patient, so EL-PFDD meetings play a crucial role in ensuring that all of our voices are heard, representing different diseases and disorders along with the necessary medications needed to treat them. The FDA wants to hear about how specific diseases, like cardiac toxicity from childhood cancer treatments, affect the daily lives of patients from a variety of stakeholders, including survivors, caregivers, other family members, medical care providers, and others. This was only the second EL-PFDD meeting that dealt with childhood cancer – the first one was about hearing loss and childhood cancer.

My participation in the EL-PFDD meeting was to record myself as I shared my story. I discussed my lifelong necessity to undergo testing and regular cardiac appointments, highlighting how protecting my heart and knowing about potential cardiac issues have affected my life. For example, I was told that my heart might not be able to withstand a pregnancy because it could put too much stress on it, especially during childbirth. Yet, hearing others' stories about their current cardiac problems, rather than potential ones like I was facing, made me wonder if I belonged with this group. Through our education about the purposes of EL-PFDD meeting, such as a focus on telling the entire story, and learning how to write what we would then record, I learned that everyone's story is different and that even though I may not have cardiac issues, I lived with the fear of them and have had to test for them at every stage of my life.

They have also altered how I have lived my life and some of the decisions I have made, especially about having children, which will be discussed further.

Peripheral Neuropathy

Peripheral neuropathy involves damage to nerves outside the brain or spinal cord and may cause the hands or feet to tingle, hurt, feel numb, or feel weak. For the longest time, I was experiencing symptoms of peripheral neuropathy, but as a child, I never told anyone because it was just one more thing that made me different, and I figured that it was just another strange thing that only affected me. For my entire life, I felt tingling and prickling sensations in my feet, and I always had to wear socks, even to bed in the middle of summer, because I had such extreme sensitivity to the feeling of the carpet beneath my feet. To this day, I still wear socks almost all the time, depending on my footwear choice, and I have a huge sock drawer full of socks of many different colors and patterns.

In addition to the sensitivity to the carpet on the bottom of my feet, I have also noticed that, at times, I experience extreme sensitivity in my hands and feet to the feeling of newspaper, bed sheets, and certain fabrics. This was just another reason I needed to wear socks to go to bed. Furthermore, I am also extremely sensitive to the cold. So, if someone stepped on my foot when it was cold, it would hurt so much more than if someone stepped on my foot when it was not cold. I have a lot of pain in my feet. My dad has this same issue, and while he has never had cancer or chemotherapy, we both have been diagnosed with neuropathy.

I also have very poor balance and coordination, which is especially evident when I am tired. When this happens, I limp and drag my right foot even more than my normal gait. This may be the result of several conditions, including peripheral neuropathy, fusion surgery, and chronic pain and weakness on the right side. If I walk too much, I get that tingling, pins and needles sensation in my feet, and then they start to go numb. This causes me to trip over myself, which is why I walk with a cane for shorter distances and use a wheelchair for longer ones. There are likely multiple reasons why I walk the way that I do, but some of the symptoms point to peripheral neuropathy as one of the potential causes.

Sinus Issues/Surgeries

One of the first long-term medical conditions that required many years of treatments and surgeries was various sinus problems. This included numerous sinus infections that lasted from weeks to months, bony polyps growing into my sinus cavities, and lots of sinus pain and pressure in my face and head. My sinus problems could not be confirmed as a late effect from neuroblastoma or any of the treatments that I received, but for several years during elementary school and junior high, I endured a lot of sinus pain, infections, and surgeries. The sinus pain was on both sides of my face, but it was worse on the right side, which, if you remember, is the side that my tumor had been located on. This is still an important issue to discuss because I had radiation to the upper chest in 1980, and it is possible that I could have been affected by scatter radiation. Scatter radiation is similar to when a droplet of water hits the floor and spreads in multiple directions, and in 1980, there was a great deal of scatter radiation that could occur.

We tried to treat the sinus problems with numerous sinus washes, a surgical procedure that involves washing out the sinus cavity. This surgery is relatively minor, and eventually, I got to the point where I could do this surgery in the doctor's office, as opposed to being put under anesthesia in the hospital. In between these relatively minor surgeries, we had to become more aggressive and perform a more invasive procedure called an intranasal ethmoidectomy – what a mouthful.

Essentially, this procedure involved my ear, nose, and throat doctor (ENT) opening up the sinus cavities and nasal pathways by breaking apart the bony polyps that had been growing into the sinuses and partially blocking them. The sinuses should simply be open spaces, and the polyps needed to be removed because they had grown and extended into the sinus cavity, causing sinus infections and immense amounts of pain and pressure.

For several years during 5th-9th grades, I had sinus surgeries every year, sometimes twice a year, alternating between the sinus washes and the intranasal ethmoidectomy surgeries. Surgeries are difficult on the body at any age, but we also had to be mindful of scar tissue forming, which could contribute to some of the pain I was experiencing. With the blessing and assistance of my local ENT doctor, we traveled across the Midwest for multiple physician consultations regarding the terrible sinus infections, the tremendous amount of facial and nasal pain, the horrendous, recurring sinus infections, and the frequent, horrific headaches that could have also been early migraines. I remember traveling with my dad to Iowa, Chicago, and Madison, Wisconsin, for various consultations with physicians who might have been able to help me.

I would try not to get too excited about these new consultations giving us a reason for, and an answer to, why I was experiencing these sinus problems. We always tried not to build it up too much because in the past, others had been unable to answer our prayers, and it always became such a massive letdown if there was nothing they could do for me. Yet, even though we told ourselves not to get excited, it was so difficult to follow our own advice. It seemed next to impossible not to get too excited, and to hope and pray that whatever new facility we were visiting, they would be able to help alleviate my sinus and head pain, as well as the need for more surgeries.

Most of the visits went reasonably well, but there was nothing new that they could offer me beyond what my home medical facility was already offering. There was one exception, however, with a very traumatizing experience when my dad and I went to Iowa to see an older doctor. This doctor, whom we shall call Dr. Ring, had answered our request for help and said that he could make a difference in the amount of pain that I was experiencing. So, we scheduled an appointment with Dr. Ring, and a short time later, my dad and I made the long drive to Iowa City.

Immediately, the atmosphere at this appointment seemed off. For example, Dr. Ring never addressed me directly; instead, he would talk over me to my dad, and any time that he had a question, he would ask my dad rather than me. Even though new doctors did not know how medically savvy I was or that I had been participating in my medical care for a long time, I was old enough to participate in my medical care when I was a teenager. And whenever he would ask a question, my dad would first look to me to answer that question so that Dr. Ring could see and know that I participated in my healthcare. Yet, that did not seem to alleviate the problem, and Dr. Ring continued to talk to my dad like I was not even in the room. Furthermore, when he did his examination, he smelled like he smoked a lot of old-fashioned pipes, which I found strange since he was an ENT.

After the examination was completed, Dr. Ring asked me to leave the room so that he could speak with my dad. I was dumbfounded and flabbergasted because I had never experienced this before. I looked at my dad, and he sort of shrugged his shoulders and indicated that I should follow the doctor's orders. So, I waited outside my exam room in a chair in a small hallway reception area. After what seemed like forever, but was likely only minutes, Dr. Ring eventually came back to get me and said, "Your dad and I sorted it all out, and we think that we have the answers to why your face and head hurt."

I was ecstatic to hear that, but for some reason, I remained guarded because something did not feel quite right. Once we got back to the room, my dad could hardly look at me. Then, Dr. Ring said, "Well, your dad and I figured it all out, and we think that everything is all in your head and that you will just grow out of it." I could not believe what I heard because during this entire journey, my greatest fear was that people would not believe that I had severe facial, head, and sinus pain. And now, I had a doctor who seized upon this fear and exploited it without, of course, even knowing it. Plus, the way Dr. Ring explained it made it seem like my dad felt the same way, and that perceived betrayal was what hurt the worst.

My dad could see how hurt I was by the doctor's announcement, and since there was not much else to say, he ushered us out of the examination room fast, directly before my anger turned to tears. As soon as we left the room, I started sobbing. We then left the ENT area, made our way to the general clinic area, and found some chairs to sit in and talk about what had happened. I started crying and trying to figure out why my dad had sided with Dr. Ring and no longer believed me. He explained that he did not feel that way at all and that Dr. Ring misspoke. He was upset that the doctor would say something like that, and he was also angry at the hurt that Dr. Ring had caused me.

We had a long drive home, requiring an hour or two of contemplation for me to process everything and truly grasp what my dad was telling me. My dad allowed me to express the anger I was holding inside, and even though I did not swear at that time, I was swearing profusely as I struggled to understand Dr. Rings' motives and as I worked through the anger that I felt from hearing and dealing with everything. We never returned to Iowa, but the effects of that trip were lasting because every once in a while, I become paranoid that someone doubts the pain that I am experiencing. That is one of the lasting results of my visit with Dr.

Ring.

Regarding the other consultations, additional medical facilities tried to help me, but they were either unable to do much more than my local medical facility, or they did not make much of a difference. For example, I had one of my sinus surgeries in Chicago. It was supposed to be just a day surgery, and we could go home after that, but it was delayed, and then it took longer to come out of the anesthesia than expected. Consequently, my dad and I had to spend an unexpected night in Chicago at the hospital. I was so upset that we had to stay in Chicago an extra night and day, which was not great for my OCD.

I was still incredibly afraid of Chicago, having spent the previous night ruminating and fixating on the crime that had happened there. I worried that it would somehow impact my dad and me during our visit for my surgery (interestingly enough, my fears were not unfounded, as all four wheel covers were stolen from the car on one of our trips to Chicago for my sinus issues). Yet, I was mostly out of it, and I could not even enjoy or open my eyes to see what was happening during my ambulance ride from the clinic to the hospital. I would have enjoyed watching some of it, but I felt very nauseous and had already vomited once. It never crossed my dad's mind or mine that we might stay the night, so we fully intended not to do so. So, without a toothbrush, change of clothes, or anything that you would pack and need in an overnight bag, my dad and I spent the night in Chicago at the hospital. We were so relieved, however, that I was fully awake and alert the next day. After post-op appointments in Chicago, we did not return for more appointments because the surgery that they did was exactly like the surgery that my local ENT could do, minus the traveling and a few other stressors.

One location we frequently returned to was a clinic at the UW Hospitals in Madison, Wisconsin, which specialized in treating headaches and pain. I was a bit apprehensive after my experience with

Dr. Ring, but this clinic assured me they could do some things that may help me, although they could not guarantee it. I liked this refreshing honesty, as opposed to the clinic claiming they could alleviate my pain while having no certainty about it. The clinic also assured me that they believed that I had pain in my sinuses and head, which I needed after many experiences with Dr. Ring. I also really liked my doctor, who first received his schooling in Croatia before coming to the United States, so he spoke with a thick accent. He was unique and wore a bolo tie, similar to what cowboys wear, which consists of a braided cord with metal tips on the ends and secured with a decorative clasp. This tie was worn instead of a regular tie, so his fashion choice set him apart from other doctors.

I had several appointments with the Madison clinic before learning about their treatment plan for me. I was informed that I needed to take one week off from school and life as I knew it, enter the hospital as an inpatient, and undergo various tests and treatments to determine what might work. At that time, I was a freshman in high school, and my goal to become valedictorian was threatened by this plan because taking ONE WEEK off from school was a significant amount of time. Yet, with the blessing of my parents, I became an inpatient in Madison for one week because it was more important to try to get rid of the sinus, facial, and head pain. I do not remember everything from my time in the hospital, but I do remember there was a lot of testing and not a lot of treatment. I also had time for schoolwork and participated in some of the activities that the hospital offered for pediatric patients.

Eventually, though, I was ready for treatment. The main treatment I had involved giving me ketamine to block the pain receptors to interrupt the pain cycle, and, therefore, ease the chronic pain. That is essentially how it was explained to us. I have read that ketamine is often used to treat severe chronic pain. It sounds easy enough, but I had a horrible reaction to the entire process. I was basically out of it, and it felt like I was having a very vivid dream. At first, I was ascending an escalator toward a very bright light, holding my cat, who had recently died. I was feeling very happy and eager to get to the bright light...Then, all of a sudden, the light and my cat disappeared, and I was plunged into darkness and felt like I was falling into hell. It was terrifying, and I wondered what I had done in my life to be entering the depths of hell.

I guess I woke up screaming and terrified from the procedure, and I was reassured that I was still alive and that I was not about to enter heaven or hell. When my "dream" switched from ascending toward the light on the escalator to plunging into darkness and hell, my blood pressure tanked, and this may have explained my rapid "dream" change and reaction to it. To this day, I still remember my feelings surrounding this incident, and it is as close to a near-death experience that I have had, and I hope never to encounter anything like it again. Also, it is unfortunate, but the ketamine treatment did not help alleviate my pain.

Thus, none of the consultations we had amounted to any change in my condition, and I continued to see my local ENT doctor. We eventually came to the point where there was nothing else that could be done for me short of a drastic surgery that involved removing my face by making an incision in the scalp. Then, they would pull my face down, like it was a rubber mask, to expose the sinus cavity and insert stomach fat into the open sinus cavities so that polyps would be unable to grow and block my cavities in the future. Finally, the surgery would end by pulling my face back up, aligning it, and sewing up the incision. This drastic, frightening surgery was an avenue that neither my family nor I wanted to pursue, so we decided to see if my sinuses would get better gradually by simply leaving them alone, as opposed to performing more surgeries and creating more scar tissue. We also tried to mitigate my risk of contracting sinus infections so often through nasal washes, extra vitamins and minerals, supplements, and more.

It took years of healing, but I eventually became free from the sinus pain. I still get terrible sinus infections that last for a long time and leave me out of commission for a bit, but they only occur about once a year. For a few years, my horrible head pain improved, too, but then I developed migraines.

Migraines

From the age of 18, I began getting migraines about once or twice a month. Until my late 30s, this condition was handled nicely by the medication I was given. I would get a migraine, take my prescription, and go back to bed for a bit. When I would wake up, I was almost always migraine-free, or they were drastically reduced. My migraine prescription worked well for me, almost magically, for many years, and I truly did not realize how blessed I was.

In my late 30s, that all changed. At that time, I began experiencing horrific migraines, but my medications no longer worked for me. I also started getting many more migraines each month, about 10-14 bad migraines, some of which would last for multiple days. The result was that I had a migraine of some sort almost every day of the month. Also, during this time, I occasionally had to go to Urgent Care and get a combination of medications to help with the pain of the migraine. Sometimes, the ER visit helped improve the pain, and occasionally, along with other methods, helped stop the migraine itself.

Due to the challenges I faced with the frequency and intensity of my migraines, I began collaborating closely with a neurologist who specialized in migraine management. Together, we began the long, arduous process of trying different medications and combinations of medications to see what would work to address my migraines. We had to be very careful with the prescriptions that we tried so that they would not adversely affect any of my existing medical issues, such as kidney disease. Due to this, we were a bit limited with some of the migraine medications that we could try.

My doctor and I tried many different medications, as well as a combination of medications. Some medications act on different receptors, which is why there are many different types of migraine medications and why a trial-and-error of medications is necessary. At the time that I was going through this medication trial, several new ones were released. Yet, since no one knew the long-term side effects or late effects of these medications, I wanted to try all of the others before we discussed trying one of the new ones, and my neurologist wholeheartedly agreed.

After years of addressing this issue, I had accrued two medications – one to take when I had or was getting a migraine and another to help with cluster migraines. We needed a solution to help prevent migraines, and we had exhausted all of the pills and injections that I was able to try with my medical conditions, with the exception of the new medications on the market. So, we decided to try something that has been used for many years to prevent migraines - Botox®. I was excited about trying Botox because it had a really good track record for helping people with difficult migraines. Everyone also wonders if you can have any extra Botox injected into your face to get rid of wrinkles. The answer to that question is no, and I think that the neurologist injecting the Botox gets asked that question multiple times a day.

For migraines, Botox is injected into the forehead, temples, back of the head, upper neck, and shoulders. You might wonder why and how this works. When you have a migraine, the body releases neurotransmitters and other molecules associated with pain. Botox (Botulinum toxin) can interfere with the transmission of neurotransmitters and other molecules. Essentially, researchers believe that Botox injections into muscles around the face, head, and neck are also taken up by the nerves and, therefore, interfere with pain from the migraine. Typically, to determine if it works, you need three or four rounds of Botox injections. Each round lasts for about three months, so it is a fairly long trial period. My first two rounds of injections went well and were uneventful. My headaches lessened by a few per month as a result, but I was eager for that third and fourth round of injections so that we could see if my migraines would be lessened to only one or two per month. After experiencing 10-14 severe migraines per month, one or two seemed like heaven. The third round of Botox was completed, and everything was uneventful.

I am uncertain about the exact timeframe following the third round of Botox when I started to experience some strange symptoms. Initially, we were unaware that the migraines were linked to these strange symptoms, which began with weakness and partial paralysis of my right arm. The lack of correlation at first was because I had similar symptoms when I had Parsonage-Turner syndrome.

Parsonage-Turner syndrome is another unique, unknown condition that I experienced during my high school years that had a large impact on my life at the time. It was a time when I was experiencing intense back pain (which I will elaborate on later in this section of the book), and I was using pain medication that caused me to sleep very deeply at night. One morning, my mother woke me up for school and noticed my speech was slurred. As I became more alert, that slurred speech eventually improved, but I did notice that I could not feel my arm – it had gone completely numb, and I was unable to move it. We decided that perhaps I had slept on my arm overnight, and since I slept so heavily, my mom told me that it was probably still asleep and that it would improve throughout the day.

That morning, I could not style my hair, put my contacts in, and put makeup on with my right arm, so my mom had to help me get ready for school. I went to school to prepare for a test, but my paralytic arm had not improved, and it did not feel like it was asleep. At my locker, I tried to grab my books and folders with my right arm, but I could not even move it, and I had to ask for assistance getting into my locker and getting to class. Although my entire arm was paralyzed and I was quite terrified because I could not move it, I was able to move my right hand and fingers, so I was able to take a test that I had been studying for and wanted to take that day. It seemed strange that my entire arm would not work, but it was a wonderful blessing that my hand and fingers worked.

I went to my local doctor after I had taken a test that day, but this doctor could not make the diagnosis and suggested that I go to the Mayo Clinic in Rochester, Minnesota. This condition first appeared on a Friday, so we made an appointment after the weekend. This meant that we had to wait an entire weekend and worry about all of the possible medical complications that could be causing my arm to be paralyzed, as well as whether or not this was a permanent situation, and other scary, terrifying, potential issues related to arm paralysis.

There was no time to rest, however, because that Saturday, the day after my arm went completely paralyzed, I had an important audition for an honors orchestra. I play the oboe, and my professional teacher and I had been preparing for this audition for months. I told my mother that I thought I could still do the audition since my fingers worked. She brought me there, styled my hair, got me dressed, and helped me put my oboe together. Then, since I was able to move my fingers, she set up my arm like we had devised the day before - she elevated my arm on pillows before securing it in a sling, ensuring it remained in the perfect position for me to play the oboe. I am sure that it looked crazy, but I was determined to go to this audition and play well. My audition went great, and I was really happy with my performance.

Following that performance, I continued to play oboe despite my arm condition. The audition and test that I had taken on Friday at school helped distract me by keeping my mind on certain goals and purposes, but in reality, I was terrified that I would never regain the use of my arm. Here I was, a high school student who just wanted to fit in and live a "normal" teenage life, but I had another HUGE medical complication that stood in the way of that desire. Also, I was completely dependent on having others help me out. I have always been very lucky and blessed to have a family that supported and helped me through everything, and this was no exception. I could not even style my own hair to get ready for the day, nor could I cut my own food to eat during meals. As a result, the independence that I craved was even more elusive because of the paralysis of my arm.

I saw a variety of doctors who conducted a barrage of tests on me, including CAT scans, MRIs, X-rays, and blood and urine tests. Most of my doctors informed me that my arm was paralyzed for unknown reasons, which left them unable to determine if I would ever regain the use of it again. We also feared that perhaps there might be a tumor in my arm and that cancer had returned. Finally, after months of appointments with various doctors, numerous blood tests, diagnostics, and other evaluations, we went to see my pediatric oncologist at the Mayo Clinic for the results of the tests.

My oncologist was *finally* able to give us a diagnosis, and we were so pleased to have an answer that had absolutely nothing to do with cancer. My paralytic right arm was diagnosed as Parsonage-Turner syndrome (PTS), also called brachial neuritis or neurologic amyotrophy. Although my condition did not follow the typical progression, PTS usually begins with severe pain and then paralysis in the shoulder, arm muscles, and joints. I do not remember any severe pain the night before or while I was sleeping, but I certainly experienced paralysis in the shoulder, arm muscles, and joints. Our doctors informed us that the condition originated with an infection settling on the brachial plexus, or a bundle of nerves in my arm, which caused the paralysis. At times, this condition can also cause aching and fever, as well as some difficulty raising the affected arm outwards and upwards, as in my case. Diagnosis of brachial neuritis includes an electromyography (EMG) and clinical history. Luckily, most cases resolve themselves, and recovery occurs within two to three years. Yet, there are also some cases, though rare, in which there was no recovery, and the damage was permanent.

Although it was wonderful to finally have a diagnosis for my arm weakness, numbness, and paralysis, I was a bit terrified to hear that the damage had the potential to be permanent, even though this is a rare complication. Yet, getting childhood cancer can be considered rare, and many of my medical conditions are also considered rare, so thinking about all of this seemed like a real possibility, and it was incredibly difficult to ponder. Furthermore, I was a freshman in high school, and at that time, thinking about the PTS lasting for two to three years seemed like such a large, substantial chunk of my life. I hoped and prayed that it would not take that long for my arm to improve so that I could try to return to my "normal" life and avoid one more medical issue.

Generally, people with this condition are advised to undergo physical therapy. There is not much else that can be done, but many doctors prescribe therapy treatments to be proactive and try to regenerate nerves and muscles in the affected arm. One main purpose of my physical therapy and exercises was to prevent atrophy of the arm muscles since they were not being used, and to see if working with those muscles and nerves could help regenerate the damaged areas at a faster rate. After my diagnosis of paralysis and several months of physical therapy, I started regaining a little mobility in my right arm. It was wonderful to finally see some improvement, but it felt like it was taking forever, and it was difficult to see such a small amount of improvement at first. However, I continued to work hard to regain the full use and mobility of my arm, and luckily, my arm paralysis only lasted for a total of nine months, as opposed to two to three years. I was one of the lucky ones because I was able to regain the full use of my arm, and my symptoms never returned.

I was in my early forties when, once again, I had problems with my right arm. It was similar to how it felt when I had PTS; however, everything felt a little different, and I was not fully paralyzed because I could lift my arm a little bit. I could not lift my arm past a certain point, though, and I had extreme weakness whenever I tried to use that arm. I also had difficulty doing things that required two hands, but in some instances, I could do them with some slight modifications. For example, styling my hair was next to impossible if I tried to do it in the "normal" way, but I could lie down and use the ground to support my hands and arms, and I could style my hair in certain ways. I went to the doctor and underwent an onslaught of testing, but doctors were stumped, and no one was able to help me determine why my arm was weak and partially paralyzed. If no one could tell me the why, it would be next to impossible to treat the arm and bring it back to normal. It was a scary time because, once again, I did not know if I would ever regain the full use of my arm.

Eventually, a neurologist put everything together and determined that my arm symptoms could be the result of Botox, especially the injections that were made into my shoulders. The doctor who administered the Botox injections was experienced and good at what she did, but because my body never seemed to follow what the medicine said it should, they thought that the injection into my shoulder went in and past the point that it was supposed to. It likely went into some of the nerves or muscles in my arm. Botox can last three to four months when it is used for wrinkles because it paralyzes the muscle, preventing movement. Yet, with complications like my arm, it can last even longer.

It was upsetting that my arm was paralyzed for the initial three to four months, especially as an adult with greater independence and responsibilities to manage. Unfortunately, the arm weakness and partial paralysis in my forties lasted more like nine to ten months. I underwent physical therapy while my arm was weak and partially paralyzed after the initial three to four months. We were hoping that this would speed up the healing process or, at the very least, help keep some of those muscles strong, even if I was unable to use them and they were incredibly weak at that time.

My arm eventually healed nicely, and I decided that since the older medications being used to treat migraines left me with such a terrible side effect, like my arm, I would try one of the newer classes of medications to see if they would help get rid of my migraines. Plus, there were virtually no other migraine medications left to try but the newer ones, and I was desperate to get rid of, or even just decrease, these migraines that were affecting and changing so much of my daily life. With my other medical challenges, I usually tried to push through. But with the migraines, it was much harder because they were all-consuming, and the pain overwhelmed my entire head.

We tried several of the new medications until we found one that prevented my migraines and continues to work today. For the first few months, my migraines decreased to between one to four per month. Eventually, in the long term, however, I now have between zero to one migraine per month. When I do get a migraine, I have a new protocol for treating it. There is a medication that I need to take as soon as I feel the migraine coming on; otherwise, it will likely not work to treat the migraine. If that is the case, or if that medicine is not working, I have an injectable that has been helping me with the pain and other symptoms when I do get a migraine. I also still take that nightly pill that helps with migraine clusters. As of 2025, things are working wonderfully, and my migraines are still at bay. It is so nice not to have to cancel something because I have a migraine or to suck it up and still work, even though my head is pounding, making it difficult to think.

Asthma, Restrictive Lung Disease

Growing up, I noticed I had difficulty breathing during strenuous activities, such as exercise and sports, especially during physical education (P.E.) class. My family and I were unaware of the reasons for this until I was older, which meant I never received any leeway or concessions during elementary, junior high, and high school P.E. classes. This meant that I still had to work just as hard as everyone else to get a decent grade in P.E. class or do some extra credit work. This was difficult for me, but vital in my quest to get a good grade and become the class valedictorian because P.E. class carries the same weight as any other class.

As I got older and grew a bit, my lung problems seemed to increase, leading to a referral to a pulmonologist, which is a doctor who focuses on diagnosing and treating respiratory system conditions. Through a series of tests, I learned that I had stress-induced asthma, typically from strenuous exercise on my body. The challenges I faced were because my right lung is approximately 50% smaller than my left lung. This is due to the tumor, radiation, and scoliosis of my spine, which makes the right side of my chest, and therefore my right lung, smaller. The radiation also caused my smaller right lung to operate at about 50% of its capacity.

We also found out that my chest wall had caved in toward my heart, which was terrifying to hear. There was discussion about possibly putting something in my chest wall to help support, hold, and shore it up to prevent it from caving in any further. Yet, that surgery would be very risky because it was extremely close to my heart, and the risk of infection would be extremely high. After the initial finding, however, I underwent further testing, and it was determined that my chest wall was stable and likely had not caved in since the initial neuroblastoma surgeries, which was a huge relief and blessing.

I have been quite lucky with my asthma – I take a daily preventive pill, and this keeps asthma attacks at bay. In the few days that I have been unable to take this medication, for whatever reason, I have noticed a difference, and I need to use my inhaler. Since my inhaler makes me shake, I try to only use it when I absolutely need it. I have been through several types of inhalers, trying to find one that does not make me shake. Typically, I only use my inhaler if I have an asthma attack or if I am having trouble breathing when I am sick with a cold or sinus infection. I have also needed to go to Urgent Care or the emergency room a few times for some nebulizer treatments, but those have only been necessary when I have been sick. Occasionally, I will wheeze quite a bit and may need to take my inhaler without being sick, but my preventive medication does a great job at preventing asthma attacks and precludes me from regularly needing to use my inhaler.

It is interesting to note that I am an oboist, which is a double-reed woodwind instrument, and I have played since I was in junior high. As I have gotten older and continue to play the oboe, my pulmonary doctor and I have noticed that my breathing has improved the more that I play. Originally, I played the flute, but the air required for playing that instrument was difficult for me to produce and maintain. However, the airflow for the oboe proved to be the perfect combination for me. A deep breath is still required, as is with any wind instrument, but for the oboe, the air is focused into a smaller area, the reed, and slowly released as it is played. It seems to work well for me, and I was told that the reason why my airflow is better is that my chest muscles have strengthened the more that I play, which, in turn, helps me with my restrictive lung disease. I am not sure if this is just something novel to me or if anyone with similar issues could play a woodwind instrument and experience something similar. Therefore, for any child having restrictive lung disease, I would advise trying to play a woodwind instrument regularly and seeing if there are any positive changes.

Adrenal Insufficiency Disease

One of the significant challenges I face is adrenal insufficiency disease, commonly referred to as AI. In addition to my chronic back pain, this condition affects me greatly and comprises a large part of why I am unable to maintain a traditional paid job. Essentially, the adrenal glands, located above the kidneys, produce several types of hormones. In my case, my body fails to produce cortisol, which is referred to as the "stress hormone." It plays a crucial role in the body's responses to stress and anxiety, along with blood pressure, blood sugar, and immune responses. In times of stress, your body is conditioned to a "fight-or-flight" response, where either your body prepares to fight whatever atypical situation is thrown at it, or your body flees and leaves the situation so that it does not have to deal with the abnormal stressor. Cortisol helps your body in times of stress, and the lack of it can wreak havoc on your life, disable your body's ability to handle stress, and cause several other unfortunate symptoms. If left untreated or not treated properly, adrenal insufficiency can also be fatal.

My cortisol levels are so low that they are practically non-existent, leading me to rely on a prescription steroid to give me the artificial levels of cortisol that I require. However, my doctors have yet to determine the underlying cause of this condition. My AI is likely not the direct result of my neuroblastoma, but it could be indirectly related. Although many cases of neuroblastoma occur in the adrenal glands, adrenal insufficiency is not directly linked to this type of childhood cancer. Furthermore, as mentioned previously, my tumor was not found in my adrenal glands or even in my abdominal cavity. AI can also occur, however, as a result of the sudden withdrawal of steroids, which are often given to treat childhood cancers and a variety of other illnesses. Many cases of adrenal insufficiency, such as my own, are typically acquired, and the cause is undetermined.

The goal of AI treatment is to take just enough steroids to function normally. If the dosage is too low, a person can feel extreme fatigue, shakiness, weakness, difficulty dealing with daily stress, prolonged recovery from even minor stressors, and light-headedness. Furthermore, additional symptoms can result, including feelings of panic, inability to handle interactions with others, angry outbursts, emotional hypersensitivity and overreactions, a tendency to be highly defensive with feelings of paranoia, flu-like symptoms, headache and all-over body aches, jitteriness, low back pain, diarrhea, and symptoms of irritable bowel syndrome (IBS).

In addition to my back pain, my adrenal insufficiency plays a huge role in how I live my everyday life and affects me when I engage in activities beyond my usual level of exertion. There are some days when I can barely leave the couch, and it is so painful and exhausting just to get up and move. This typically occurs the day after I have engaged in activities outside of the house beyond my routine daily life. It can also occur if I have been home, but I have had multiple virtual meetings throughout the day. The good news is that after I have had difficult days, I can still do some work on my laptop while lying down and without leaving the couch. I do not always feel like I am doing my best work during this time, but at least I can get some work accomplished.

For me, the most challenging symptom of adrenal insufficiency is undoubtedly the fatigue. Although I have also been diagnosed with chronic fatigue syndrome and experience insomnia, I think that a great deal of my fatigue comes from my AI. On days when I do not take enough steroids, simply moving from one end of the house to the other feels like a major achievement. Additionally, there are times when my fatigue is so overwhelming that I experience intense nausea. On those days, I need to take more steroids than my base dose. However, it is a balancing act because the goal is to take the least amount of steroids possible while still being able to function normally and not experience symptoms. When I have an extremely busy day, whether it be physically, emotionally, or mentally, I typically need to take a stress dose of steroids. A stress dose simply involves taking more than my routine dose of steroids to help my body get through the extra stress of a busy, taxing day. For surgeries, for example, my doctors and I typically double my usual dose, and I also get a bolus, or a large number of steroids injected into my IV at one time during surgery. I would also need extra steroids if I were unconscious or vomiting. If this were the case, I would need an injection of steroids before being taken to the hospital to be monitored. My body must have extra levels of steroids during surgeries, when I am sick, and during times of extra stress, and I wear a medical bracelet stating that I have AI and need steroids. In an emergency, the lack of extra steroids could be fatal or put me into an adrenal coma.

Since I have become more active with my nonprofits and writing this book, I have had to take more than my base dose of steroids on a fairly regular basis. This allows me the opportunity to get things done, but it is also hard on my body because I am continually taking more steroids regularly rather than taking my usual base dose. I only permit myself to rest when it is absolutely necessary, which amounts to once or twice per week. This "rest" usually consists of sleeping for the majority of the day and not doing much of anything. However, I tend to be quite critical of myself, believing that I should contribute to childhood cancer initiatives and at least one of my nonprofit organizations every single day.

There are certainly days when I feel like my life is just fading away, especially during moments when I can only lie on the couch, staring blankly at the television. Throughout high school and college, I led a very hectic life with an action-packed schedule of music and academics. It is incredibly challenging to reflect on my past and the energy that I once had, and compare it to how I am today. Very few people understand this condition and how it affects me. When I am invited to events, and I am unable to go, it is very difficult for me to decline and try to explain the situation. I also am the type of person who constantly agonizes and worries over what other people think of me, and those feelings are working overtime when my AI is active and getting in the way of life.

Dealing with my various medical conditions can turn a regular day into a difficult one. Yet, when a special event is happening, making it through the day can become exceptionally tough, often leaving me in need of several days to recuperate. It can be challenging for others to grasp the nature of my condition and why participating in a single event feels so different from attending my childhood cancer conferences that span multiple days. When I attend these multi-day conferences, I take a high dose of steroids throughout my attendance. I am only able to sustain this for five to seven days maximum, and then my body demands rest time. Once I get home, it takes several days of sleeping and not doing anything to recover from the conference or event.

There have been several occasions in my life when I've faced an adrenal crisis. Before my diagnosis of adrenal insufficiency (AI), we lacked a specific name for the condition. However, it always began in the same way. I would fall asleep and remain in a near-unconscious state for extended periods. This typically occurred after experiencing a medical issue or during particularly hectic times when I struggled to find any rest. For example, after I had the ketamine dose in Madison to try to stop the pain cycle of sinus and facial pain, along with my headaches, we were preparing to go home the following day, and I kept falling asleep. My mom was driving us home, and she was hoping that I could help her with the directions for getting back on the interstate, but I kept falling asleep. Shortly into our journey, she bought us sub sandwiches because we had not eaten lunch, and it was a bit too early for supper. She was also hoping that eating would keep me awake. It did not. I kept falling asleep while I was eating, and I would even fall asleep with the sub on the way to my mouth. I ended up wearing a blanket of shredded lettuce, and my mom realized that nothing was working to keep me awake.

My mom was a bit terrified, but she let me sleep until we got home. Once home, my mother attempted additional efforts to keep me awake. She tried to see if I would practice the piano, but I fell asleep on the keys. She also tried to see if I could start writing some of the many "Thank You" notes that I owed friends and family who remembered me being in the Madison hospital for one week. The result was my writing some nonsensical messages and wasting cards.

The next day, my pediatrician insisted on seeing me, and I was so out of it that I wore some ugly pajamas to the appointment. The medical staff and my doctor quickly evaluated me and determined that I belonged in the hospital. We were very scared regarding the potential causes of this issue, and thus far, all tests had returned negative results. However, the general consensus was that I might have meningitis. Regardless, I was scared, yet barely awake to fully process anything.

Luckily, my dad recalled that I had gone through a similar experience before, during which I was prescribed steroids that proved effective. So, the doctors administered steroids, and I quickly returned to my normal self after taking the medication and enjoying a restful night's sleep. At that moment, we didn't fully understand why this approach worked for me, but we were all grateful that I was back to my usual self and that I did not have meningitis.

More than 30 years after this happened, I experienced a few adrenal crises with my husband, Troy. My busy schedule was typically the cause of the crisis, along with some type of medical issue, and it always started with me being extremely tired and sleeping all the time. I recall a particular instance when, throughout the night and into the early morning, Troy attempted unsuccessfully to wake me. Most of the time, he didn't manage to do so, but I do remember briefly waking a few times, even if just for seconds or minutes. I also remember that Troy succeeded in getting me out of bed to use the bathroom, brush my teeth, and wash my face, but beyond that, his efforts fell short. I would not stay awake, and I am not exactly sure that saying I was "asleep" is accurate. I was pretty much unresponsive, and perhaps you could say unconscious. I did not know this at the time, but Troy was so worried about me that he decided to sleep in the recliner because I was asleep on the couch. He did not sleep well and repeatedly tried to wake me up. He even put me in the shower and turned on the water at an extremely cold temperature. It did temporarily "wake me up," and I think that I got upset with Troy for doing that to me. However, I was back to being unresponsive shortly after, and the only part of this incident that I do remember is the blast of cold water.

Eventually, we had to go to the emergency room to address the adrenal crisis that started at home, as I required an infusion of steroids to help me recover. I know that Troy tried so hard to wake me and that he was profoundly worried about me. I felt just awful that I put him through this entire situation. However, my body went into an adrenal crisis, and I needed the infusion to remain awake and conscious. If I do not receive the steroids my body needs, I risk entering an adrenal coma, which could ultimately lead to death. It was evident that I was experiencing an adrenal crisis because my system was so depressed, yet my heart rate was high. In addition, I was beyond the point of exhaustion, and I was unresponsive, tired, and essentially unconscious. I was also experiencing weakness, dizziness, disorientation, and low blood pressure. These are all symptoms of an adrenal crisis, but other symptoms that I had not experienced were muscle aches, nausea, vomiting, and diarrhea. Finally, hypoglycemia, hyperpigmentation, dehydration, and weight loss are also symptoms of an adrenal crisis, yet I do not typically experience them during an adrenal crisis.

Another time when I experienced an adrenal crisis was during a minor surgery. As with all my surgical procedures, I dedicated significant effort to compiling a list of tasks I wanted to complete beforehand. This included not only finishing work for my nonprofits but also tackling various chores around the house. This approach was consistent with my previous surgeries. Additionally, I usually struggle to sleep the night before surgery because I have so much to accomplish and need to wake up early. I took a stress dose of steroids, and I received a bolus of steroids during the surgery, which is typical for me whenever I have major or minor surgery. Yet, for some reason, this time was different, and after the surgery, the nurse had me sit up on the side of the bed and then stand. I promptly fainted. Luckily, my husband and the nurse caught me, and things moved awfully fast after that. I was put back into bed, and tests were conducted. They noticed that my blood pressure was low and my heart rate was high, which was one of the symptoms of adrenal insufficiency. I slept a lot during this time and did not remember much, but someone mentioned my AI, and a medical professional put it together that I was likely experiencing an adrenal crisis. More steroids were given to me, and almost instantaneously, I reawakened.

As you have read, I manage my adrenal insufficiency disease through a regimen of oral tablets. On typical days with minimal activity, I take a standard base dose of medication, and on more demanding days filled with activity, I can take higher doses of steroids. Around my forties, however, I was also introduced to another treatment option, steroid injections. At times when I may be unconscious, or at times when I cannot keep oral steroids down, either Troy or I can give myself an injection. We received instructions on administering an injection at the endocrinologist's office using faux skin, but we have not had to put this into practice yet. If we ever do have to give me an injection, we would then need to immediately call the ambulance or go to the emergency room so that I could be examined or monitored.

Thyroid Nodules and Hypothyroidism

Since I had radiation to the chest in the early 80s, scatter radiation was prominent, and it was highly possible that the thyroid gland was within that area. In addition to the radiation, I had certain types of chemotherapy medications that put me at a much greater risk of getting thyroid cancer as a secondary cancer. In 2011 and 2012, I underwent thyroid cancer scares, and the surgery to remove my thyroid and the nodules attached to it occurred in October 2012. This was before my work with childhood cancer nonprofits, including my survivorship research, and I did not know at that time that thyroid cancer was a common secondary cancer from the treatments that I had undergone for childhood cancer.

Initially, I began experiencing occasional problems swallowing, during which I would be unable to swallow whatever saliva, food, or liquid was in my mouth at that time. There seemed to be no clear cause for this issue, but it was frustrating when it happened because I would try to swallow repeatedly, but it felt like something was blocking me from being able to do so. In addition, at times, I had increased pain and pressure in my neck. I also experienced some voice hoarseness, and as a soprano singer, this could limit how high I could sing. Typically, I would only experience similar voice hoarseness if I had a cold or a sinus infection. Even though I had gastroesophageal reflux disease (GERD), my singing was not usually affected, and I could hit my usual high notes with little to no difficulty. However, throughout 2012, as some of my thyroid nodules doubled in size, I was a little panicked about losing some of my high-pitched range when singing.

It was even more troubling when I visited the endocrinologist, and just like many times before, he started feeling and palpating my neck. I noticed that he spent a little too long feeling my neck, and I could see the inquisitive look on his face. I asked what was wrong because I could tell there was something off. It was written all over my doctor's face. He informed me that my thyroid felt swollen, and I asked what that meant. It was difficult to feel exactly what was going on with my thyroid, but the doctor suspected that it was extra-large because there were multiple large nodules attached to it.

I had scans that confirmed what the doctor suspected - I had multiple large nodules attached to my thyroid gland, or a multinodular goiter. Furthermore, my trachea was slightly pushed off to the right, which could have been from the original tumor pushing it aside, from the nodules themselves, or a combination of the two. All of this was viewed on a CT scan that was conducted in July 2011, but the nodules dated all the way back to a thoracic CT scan in January 2007. Yet, no one had seen that information on the January 2007 CT scan, so we were not informed of any irregularities until I began to experience symptoms in early 2011 and 2012, when the situation had intensified significantly.

Given the significant enlargement of my thyroid gland due to the nodules, along with my history of chest radiation and the symptoms I was experiencing, a thyroidectomy was inevitable. Whether the nodules were cancerous or non-cancerous did not factor into that decision because the thyroid gland simply needed to be removed for me to be able to swallow regularly again and to contain my thyroid, which was rather large from the nodules. No matter what, it was important to perform a biopsy to determine whether or not the nodules were cancerous. If cancerous, this information would guide us on the treatments I would require to cure this secondary cancer. If it were non-cancerous, we knew that the treatment would end with the removal of the thyroid gland.

In late 2011, I had an ultrasound to measure nodules and several biopsies to test for cancer. This was quite a painful process, and I cannot remember exactly how many biopsies were needed, but they wanted to biopsy each nodule, some in multiple places, so that they could be sure that they were testing every nodule. Shortly after the biopsies were completed, my neck started swelling and bruising spectacularly, and it was a bit painful to move my head and neck. Yet, the biopsies were necessary, and after what seemed like a very long wait, they told us that the growing nodules that encapsulated my thyroid gland were NON-cancerous.

In July 2012, I underwent another ultrasound to update the previous one. During the manual examination, it appeared that the right lobe of the thyroid might have been slightly smaller; however, the overall size of the thyroid gland had increased, particularly on the left side. The report indicated that there was a nodule in the mid lobe measuring 2.2 cm, a nodule in the right lower lobe measuring 1 cm, a nodule in the left upper lobe measuring 2.6 cm, a nodule in the left lower lobe measuring 4.7 cm, and a nodule in the isthmus measuring 1 cm. Two of the nodules had more than doubled in size since the last measurements were taken; one had decreased slightly in size, and the other two nodules remained approximately the same size.

I had surgery to remove my thyroid and all of the nodules attached to it, and I vividly remember that this was the last time that I took Versed before surgery. Now, I specifically ask not to have this medication before surgery. The purpose of taking it is to help a patient relax before surgery, but it can also cause a patient to forget about what is happening and fall asleep. In my case, I was given Versed before my thyroidectomy, and apparently, I began talking about a lot of things that I just do not fully remember.

After surgery, when I did not even remember being brought to the surgical suite, I asked my husband and parents if I looked or sounded like an idiot during this time. Instead of reassuring me that I had not, they looked at each other and said, "Maybe you did a little bit." I was shocked and mortified, and I asked them what I said to sound so ridiculous. They told me that when the surgeon came to visit, I kept saying that I wanted to see the thyroid gland after it had been removed because I had never seen one before. When I was informed that this was not possible, I pressed on and asked why. It was explained that the thyroid was so large and had so many large nodules that it needed to be taken out in multiple pieces. Instead of letting it go, I asked why the pieces of the thyroid gland could not be "thoughtfully arranged" after they had been removed. I never got an answer on that one because my family finally got me to stop talking about this, and the surgeon never addressed it again!

Given the complications that I can have after surgery because of all of my preexisting conditions and late effects from my cancer and its treatments, this was a fairly easy surgery. I had no trouble with my adrenal insufficiency disease. They had me stay overnight as a precaution, but I had no complications. When I woke up from anesthesia, I could barely tell where the incision had been made to remove my thyroid – the surgeon did a brilliant job of stitching up the opening, and it just looked like a natural part of my neck. More than a decade later, this is one scar that I cannot even see or show off.

As a result of that surgery, I have acquired hypothyroidism, which essentially means that because I no longer have a thyroid gland, I no longer produce thyroid hormones. I will have this condition for the rest of my life, but luckily, I can take an oral synthetic thyroid hormone to replace what my thyroid would have produced. Without taking this medication, or if the thyroid is underactive, the symptoms of hypothyroidism include fatigue, weight gain, difficulty tolerating cold, joint and muscle pain, dry skin, dry and thinning hair, heavy or irregular menstrual periods and fertility problems, slowed heart rate, and depression. So, it is important to take my medication to avoid dealing with these difficult symptoms. On the other hand, there are times when I could also experience hyperthyroidism (receiving too much of the thyroid hormone). This manifests in symptoms such as weight loss, hand tremors, rapid and irregular heartbeat, heart palpitations, increased hunger, anxiety and irritability, sweating and sensitivity to heat, fatigue, muscle weakness, sleep problems, and fine and brittle hair. Taking the medication is not an exact science, so that is why it is important to get regular thyroid tests to determine if the thyroid levels are underactive, overactive, or just right.

Stage 3 Kidney Disease

Before contracting chronic kidney disease (CKD) and experiencing some of the complications that can arise as chronic kidney disease progresses, I never really thought about everything that the kidneys can impact. CKD, however, can affect almost every part of the body. The main responsibility of the kidneys is to filter waste and excess fluids from the blood, which then leaves the body through urine. Treatment for CKD involves slowing down the progression of kidney damage, typically by controlling the cause of the kidney disease if it is known. The thought is that my kidneys might have been damaged by chemotherapy. Additionally, in the 1990s and early 2000s, I tried a series of NSAIDs, or non-steroidal anti-inflammatory drugs, to see if we could find something to help with my chronic, agonizing back pain. We did not find anything that helped in a significant way, and it is possible that all of those NSAID trials damaged my kidneys. So, either my kidneys were damaged by chemotherapy treatments, or they were damaged by a series of NSAIDs that I took for my chronic pain.

Even if you treat and slow down the progression of kidney damage by controlling the cause, you may not stop kidney disease from progressing. CKD can sometimes progress to end-stage kidney failure, which is fatal unless there is dialysis, which artificially filters your urine, or a kidney transplant. There are several stages of CKD, which can be measured in two ways, using a blood test called the glomerular filtration rate (GFR), which is calculated by how much your body is filtering certain waste products, such as creatinine. Second, CKD can be measured through a urine test, which examines the urine albumin to creatinine ratio, or the amount of protein in the urine, indicating how much the kidneys are leaking protein and not filtering properly. I typically undergo regular blood tests to measure the amount of creatinine in my blood, as well as the estimated GFR or eGFR.

The measurement of the eGFR and the stage of kidney disease are depicted below:

- eGFR of 90 or higher for at least three months is in the normal range and is considered Stage 1.
- eGFR of 60 -89 for at least three months may mean early-stage kidney disease, or Stage 2.
- eGFR of 15 -59 for at least three months may mean kidney disease. Stage 3a is 45-59, Stage 3b is 30-44, and Stage 4 kidney disease has an eGFR of 15-29.
- eGFR below 15 for at least three months may mean kidney failure, and this is considered Stage 5.

The signs and symptoms depend on how advanced the CKD is in the body, and these can include nausea, vomiting, and a loss of appetite. A person can also feel fatigue and weakness, develop sleep problems, and have decreased mental sharpness. A person may urinate more than or less than normal, or they may have muscle cramps, swelling of the feet and ankles, fluid retention, and/or dry, itchy skin. Finally, CKD can cause hypertension (high blood pressure), shortness of breath from fluid buildup in the lungs, and chest pains from fluid buildup around the lining of the heart.

In addition to filtering and removing extra water and natural waste products from the body, the kidneys also assist in balancing important minerals in the body, help create red blood cells, maintain a healthy blood pressure, and keep bones strong and healthy. The treatment for CKD involves managing the cause of it, if known, and taking steps to slow down the progression.. In addition, it is important to lower the risk of cardiovascular disease, such as a heart attack or stroke. Finally, treating CKD involves treating all of the complications that may result from medications, nutrition, and lifestyle recommendations.

My complications are common ones associated with kidney disease, and they can continue to worsen if the disease progresses. Currently, if you examine the eGFR explanation aforementioned, my CKD hovers between Stage 3a and 3b. Due to this, I have several complications from CKD, and the remainder of this section examines several of the complications that I currently have or had, including the symptoms and how they are treated.

Chronic Anemia:

Anemia, a common complication of CKD, is a condition where the blood has lower levels of red blood cells or hemoglobin. Hemoglobin is an iron-rich protein that allows red blood cells to carry oxygen throughout the body. This condition continues to worsen as CKD progresses, and the result is that certain parts of the body may not get enough oxygen to work properly.

Sometimes, there have been no symptoms when I have been anemic, and other times, there have been some severe symptoms. Typically, for anemia, I feel quite fatigued, weak, and lightheaded, but sometimes those symptoms will be accompanied by headaches, shortness of breath, and heart palpitations.

During lab tests that assess various kidney-related levels, I usually find my red blood cell count to be low, while my hemoglobin levels tend to be at the lower end of the normal range or slightly below it. As CKD progresses, these levels will typically get worse. There have been times, however, when I have needed a little medical intervention to help me get past the anemia. For example, over ten years ago, I needed iron transfusions because I was so anemic. Luckily, these transfusions worked for me, and after the recommended dosage, I have not needed any more of these transfusions. I also had a minor surgery that ended up having some major complications. I ended up bleeding a lot from the surgery, and my hemoglobin got so low that I needed a blood transfusion. Overall, however, I have been quite lucky bouncing back from anemia with some simple, gentle iron pills, which are better for a sensitive stomach.

Fluid Retention:

Within the last few years, I have experienced fluid retention and swelling in my legs and feet. This swelling in the body, also known as edema, can be quite common in CKD because the kidneys are having trouble removing excess fluid from the body. This fluid retention or edema can affect the arms, hands, and face, although I do not experience much fluid retention in these areas at this time. I do have some swelling on a daily basis if I have had a bit more physical activity that day or the previous day. Yet, I have really noticed this swelling and fluid retention whenever I am traveling, including after an airplane flight and throughout the duration of the trip, and then every day of the conference after that. I used to only start retaining fluids after being active for several days, but then it would dissipate quite quickly. However, it has gotten so bad that I need to wear compression stockings whenever I take a trip, and those just are not sexy! I also take a diuretic three times a week to help with the minor fluid retention that I experience daily.

Retaining fluid and ending up looking like the Michelin man or the large version of Eddie Murphy in The Nutty Professor does not necessarily hurt; it is just uncomfortable and pretty alarming to see my body swell that much. When I reach a certain amount of fluid retention, my legs get pretty stiff, and it can be quite difficult to walk. I do walk with a cane in my everyday life, and I am intensely grateful to have it when my legs and feet are retaining fluid.

It is also important to avoid sodium to help with fluid retention and edema. This is so difficult for me because I have a very sensitive stomach and do not typically indulge in a lot of spices or seasoning. I have always said that salt is my favorite spice! Yet, I have had to learn restraint with using salt, and now I use a well-known seasoning blend that is quite delicious and helps me avoid using salt altogether at times. Other ways to help prevent fluid retention and edema are to monitor your blood pressure, weigh yourself daily, and decrease fluid intake.

Do you know all those jokes about cankles? Yes, they do apply to me when I am traveling or have increased activity. However, I am doing the best that I can to deal with fluid retention and to still live a fulfilling life by attending conferences, advocating for childhood cancer, meeting patients, families, and survivors, and talking with and learning from other nonprofit organizations.

<u>Vitamin D Deficiency</u>:

In February 2005, I had an injury that gave me a horrific amount of extra pain, and that ultimately made my chronic back pain worse. It also took what seemed like forever to diagnose. One night, I fell out of bed onto my butt or my sacrum, which is the triangle-shaped bone at the end of the spine. The next day and for weeks after, I could hardly walk because it hurt to put pressure and weight on the right side. I also could not sit for very long because I would get unbearable pain on the right side, so I had to balance all of my weight on the left side until it would get tired and sore, and I could no longer do it.

I waited several days, hoping that the pain would lessen, but it did not get any better, and I eventually went to multiple doctors. For weeks, I endured countless tests, including a CT scan, X-rays, two MRI scans, blood and urine tests, and a bone density test. At first, the tests were inconclusive, and nothing yielded any results. It was getting frustrating because I could hardly walk, and at the time, I was working eight-hour workdays, which was big for me because I was already dealing with chronic pain. After three weeks of waiting for test results that yielded nothing, I had a bone scan and a second MRI, which revealed a bone fracture, or break, in my sacrum. Due to my spinal fusion, this area of my body took the entire impact of my fall and fractured on impact.

This was the first bone that I had ever broken, which was unfortunate, but it was also a relief to know that the intense pain that I was feeling had a legitimate cause. The doctor was amazed, as well, with how strong I was in dealing with the pain, and she promptly set me up with crutches, bed rest, and increased pain medications. I took a leave of unpaid absence from work (unpaid because my employment date with my company had been in dispute. My company had forced me to start working for them through a temporary agency for what they stated would be at least three months, but it turned out to be a lot more than that. Although I requested multiple times to have my employment changed over to the actual company, that date was delayed multiple times through no fault of my own. Unfortunately, when my injury occurred, I was right on the bubble to qualify for paid FMLA leave.)

The healing process for the actual fracture took over one full year. However, I have arthritis and pain in the area where I fractured my sacrum, and now it comprises part of my chronic pain. Further, another important component of the healing process was determining why a young woman in her mid-twenties would fracture a bone by simply falling out of bed. This, of course, meant additional rounds of testing to determine the causes. We discovered that I had low levels of vitamin D, which is a vitamin that aids the body in the absorption of calcium. So, I was getting plenty of calcium in my body, but without adequate levels of vitamin D, my body was not able to use that calcium, resulting in weakened bones. To treat this condition, my doctor prescribed a HUGE amount of vitamin D to take once a week for the rest of my life.

This condition may or may not have been a result of my CKD because I had chronically low levels of vitamin D before I was officially diagnosed. However, I could have had undiagnosed CKD, or perhaps this condition was independent of or in addition to something else. Whatever the case, the kidneys play a significant part in the regulation and metabolism of vitamin D. Specifically, the kidneys produce an enzyme that is required to turn inactive vitamin D into its active form. Yet, when this enzyme is decreased, it can lead to reduced levels of active or usable vitamin D, which then causes the body to absorb less calcium.

Osteopenia:

Osteopenia is characterized by mild bone thinning, loss, and weakening of the bone. It may serve as a precursor to osteoporosis, a condition marked by decreased bone mineral density and mass, along with changes in bone structure and strength. These factors can elevate the risk of fractures. Often referred to as the silent killer, osteoporosis can remain undetected until a problem arises or testing is conducted. Both osteopenia and osteoporosis can result from a variety of factors, including hormonal, genetic, dietary, age-related, and lifestyle influences.

Following my sacral fracture, my doctors briefly contemplated prescribing osteoporosis medication; however, there was a lack of long-term studies regarding its use. Generally, this medication was not recommended for women in their mid to late twenties, which was my age at the time of the fracture. Additionally, my condition improved after I began taking extra vitamin D, making the osteoporosis medication unnecessary. Nevertheless, I continue to have regular bone density tests to ensure my bones are not thinning too quickly. This is important as rapid thinning can be a common late effect for childhood cancer survivors.

Secondary Hyperparathyroidism:

The parathyroid glands, consisting of four small glands located near the thyroid gland, release the parathyroid hormone, which controls the amount of calcium in your blood and bones. If there is little calcium in the blood and bones, the parathyroid gland releases extra parathyroid hormones, and vice versa. When these glands become enlarged and result in a high blood level of the parathyroid hormone, the result is secondary hyperparathyroidism.

When a patient has kidney disease, as is in my case, there are several reasons why this can happen, such as high phosphorus levels in the blood, the kidneys not making active vitamin D (which is needed to absorb calcium), and low blood calcium levels. In my case, my kidneys do not make active vitamin D, which is needed to absorb the calcium that the body is taking in. This means that this secondary hyperparathyroidism can cause a buildup of calcium in tissues and organs, like the heart and blood vessels, and it can cause bone disease. There is an intricate balance to give the body enough calcium but not too much. My secondary hyperparathyroidism is treated by medications and supplements, as well as controlling the phosphorus levels in the blood. Additional treatments can include surgery, but thankfully, that has not been necessary in my case.

Chronic Hypokalemia:

Potassium is a necessary mineral because it conducts electricity throughout the body, which keeps the heart beating regularly and muscles functioning properly. When there is not enough potassium in the body and the levels become very low, like mine, one could experience symptoms like muscle twitches, muscle cramps, faintness, and low blood pressure. The muscle cramps are certainly no joke, and they can be pretty painful and intense. I just have to try to calmly breathe through the muscle cramps. One could also experience abnormal heart rhythms, but luckily, I have not experienced any symptoms directly related to my heart.

To treat hypokalemia, I take a potassium supplement several times a day. I have also been advised to eat potassium-rich foods, but many of the options are foods that I cannot eat because of a GI disorder that I have, which we will discuss later. I do the best that I can, but recently, I have had to increase the dosage of prescription potassium that I need to take daily because my levels have been chronically low again.

Chronic Hypomagnesemia:

In addition to chronically low potassium, I have chronically low magnesium, which often goes together with low potassium. I need to take a prescription-strength supplement of magnesium as well. Magnesium is important because it is typically found in the bones and soft tissues, and a small amount is found in the blood. At times, low levels of magnesium may simply mean that more magnesium needs to be ingested. With kidney disease, however, hypomagnesemia occurs when too much magnesium is lost through the kidneys.

As you may have noticed, I deal with multiple medical conditions, and their symptoms can overlap, making it challenging to determine which symptom belongs to which condition. For instance, I experience muscle cramps due to both low potassium and low magnesium, along with hand tremors and spasms. Additional symptoms of low magnesium include weakness, fatigue, nausea, vomiting, and loss of appetite; however, these can also be associated with various other conditions. Generally, since low magnesium and low potassium often occur simultaneously, distinguishing the symptoms of each condition becomes quite complex.

Chronic Hypophosphatemia:

If you are following the pattern, you will already know that hypophosphatemia means a low level of phosphate in the blood. Essentially, phosphate contains the mineral phosphorus, which is needed to help the body build and repair bones and teeth; help nerves function; and make your muscles tighten. The majority of the body's phosphorus, contained in phosphate, is found in the body's bones.

Mild hypophosphatemia does not have any signs or symptoms, but more severe levels can cause muscle and bone pain, muscle weakness, altered mental status such as confusion or irritability, altered mental status, respiratory or heart failure, numbness, seizures, coma, and death, but only in the most extreme cases. To be honest, I am not sure if I have experienced muscle and bone pain or severe muscle weakness from this condition because, again, these are some of the symptoms that I have for my other conditions. However, my kidney doctor and I are treating this condition by taking prescription-strength supplements.

Finally, there are several causes of hypophosphatemia, and for me, it is hard to discern which one is responsible. High levels of hyperparathyroidism can cause hypophosphatemia, as well as hypokalemia and hypomagnesemia. Vitamin D deficiency can also cause low levels of phosphates, so it is difficult to discern which condition contributed to the hypophosphatemia.

Hypertension:

My blood pressure used to be perfect, but eventually, we discovered that my blood pressure became quite high. Days before my 44th birthday in 2023, I was given the gift of multiple blood pressure medications. Although it is normal for a person's blood pressure to rise and fall throughout the day, it cannot be high for too long because it can damage the heart and cause various health problems.

The second leading cause of kidney failure in the U.S. is uncontrolled high blood pressure. This causes the blood vessels in your kidneys to narrow, reducing blood flow and stopping the kidneys from working efficiently and effectively. The kidneys are unable to remove all wastes and extra fluids from the body. Extra fluid in the blood vessels can increase blood pressure even more, so it is a vicious cycle that causes more and more damage and can lead to kidney failure. Damaged kidneys do not filter blood well and fail to regulate blood pressure. Therefore, it is of the utmost importance to regularly check and monitor a person's blood pressure and take steps to keep it as low as possible.

Gastrointestinal (GI) Issues

I have multiple GI issues that are intertwined, and it can be difficult to tell where one ends and the other begins. This, in part, is due to the numerous medical issues that I have, as well as the medications that I take to address those issues. Although the prescriptions that I take help me with some of my medical conditions, they are also powerful enough to cause or worsen various GI issues. It is a balancing act, and I have to make daily decisions about which prescriptions I take each day while keeping in mind the possible repercussions of these decisions.

Acid Reflux and Gastroesophageal Reflux Disease (GERD):

The first GI issue that emerged was heartburn, or acid reflux, which occurs when the acid from the stomach gets backed up into the esophagus and even the throat. The acid irritates the esophagus and the throat, causing burning stomach and chest pain, also called heartburn. Almost everyone has felt some form of heartburn in their lives, so acid reflux is quite common and is not anything to worry about on its own.

Chronic acid reflux, however, can damage tissues and affect a person's quality of life. Gastroesophageal reflux disease (GERD) is the medical term used to describe chronic acid reflux, which means that the condition occurs at least twice a week over several weeks. Acid Reflux is caused by temporary conditions, but GERD means that the mechanisms that are supposed to keep acid out of your esophagus are not working properly. Furthermore, GERD is also a common condition, affecting about 20% of adults in the United States and 10% of children. In addition to a burning feeling or the sour taste of acid, some of the symptoms of GERD include nausea, a sore throat, noncardiac-related chest pain, and asthma-like symptoms. I have experienced all of these symptoms and continue to do so on bad days. There are a variety of over-the-counter medications that can be used to treat acid reflux, and several prescription medications to treat GERD. For severe cases of GERD that are resistant to other treatments, there are also surgical options. Patients can also try various natural remedies at home. I take a daily preventative medication twice a day, which helps lessen the symptoms of GERD, and on some days, I have no symptoms at all!

Irritable Bowel Syndrome:

My first abdominal pain began in the early 2000s when I was about 20 years old, and I was having bad stomach pains that were different than what I had experienced through GERD or any other medical condition up to that point. The pain would especially worsen whenever I would eat, and then I would either get diarrhea or constipation.

Throughout several years, my doctors put me through a series of tests to rule out certain issues and to hopefully determine the problem. I had blood tests, as well as an ultrasound, an MRI, a CT Scan, and an X-ray, to try and make sure there was nothing abnormal. The worst tests I had, however, were an endoscopy and a colonoscopy. An endoscopy is a test where a small tubular camera is placed down a patient's throat to check the upper part of the digestive tract, and a colonoscopy is where the camera is inserted into a patient's anus to look at the lower part of the digestive tract. I have no problem with the endoscopy... it is the colonoscopy that is the source of a LOT of grief!

With both of the tests, you are essentially put to sleep, so the tests themselves are not the problem. The problem is the preparation for the colonoscopy, which involves drinking a TON of a horrible-tasting substance and refraining from eating or drinking anything that is not clear. The goal is to clear out the colon so that when the test is performed, there is a clear view of the lower digestive tract. I have had the test done many times, but when I had it for the first time, I threw up the entire time that I tried to drink the horrible concoction. I could only drink about half of what I was supposed to drink, and from the lack of food for a few days, I got a horrible headache and felt horrendous. Due to this experience, I developed a horrible gag reflex that kicks in and does not allow me to eat or drink anything unfavorable. Furthermore, I had to fast for a few days longer than usual, and that made things worse. In the end, the test showed nothing, which was even more frustrating to me.

One time, an endoscopy revealed that I had an ulcer that was healing, but most of the time, the tests did not reveal much in the form of a diagnosis for why my stomach felt so bad. The tests did not reveal much in the form of a diagnosis for my stomach issues at that time, so I was diagnosed with irritable bowel syndrome, which at that time was sort of a catch-all diagnosis. Irritable bowel syndrome involves pain in the abdominal area, as well as changes in bowel movements, such as diarrhea, constipation, or, in my case, both. The diarrhea and constipation would ebb and flow, typically according to the amount of opioids that I was taking for my chronic back pain, which will be discussed soon. Whether I was experiencing diarrhea or constipation, there were times when I would be doubled over in pain. Yet, little did we know that there were other factors at play.

Clostridium difficile (C.diff) infection:

In February 2008, I started experiencing diarrhea... ALL THE TIME. I started to lose a tremendous amount of weight, so my doctors advised me to try taking Immodium AD before each meal to attempt to combat the diarrhea, and occasionally, that does help. However, I continued experiencing diarrhea after everything that I ate. To try and help the problem, I researched probiotics, which are bacteria in your stomach that your body naturally produces, but there are times when your body does not produce enough. Thus, you can supplement them with over-the-counter probiotics, which I tried taking to see if it would help. Unfortunately, they did not affect me much.

Over two years, I lost more than 40 pounds because of the diarrhea, and although it was nice to lose weight, this was a miserable way of doing it! I went through a barrage of tests, and my doctor informed me that I had C.diff and that I may have had it on and off for two years, resulting in severe weight loss. C.diff is a bacteria that can cause diarrhea and life-threatening colitis or inflammation of the colon. Typically, it affects older adults or people from a long-term care facility, but it can also affect anyone in a health care facility. This is because C. diff is naturally present in the colon, but it is kept at bay and regulated by other bacteria. When taking an antibiotic, however, you are not only killing the bacteria causing the sickness, but you may also be affecting the balance of C.diff in the stomach because there are fewer bacteria to regulate these levels. The result is that they can massively grow and cause a C.diff infection, which coincidentally is treated with a specific antibiotic. I was treated for this infection multiple times because I kept having the infection over and over, but I was finally infection-free after two years, a few rounds of antibiotics, and the loss of 40 pounds.

Appendicitis:

Over the summer of 2008, I began having extremely localized and intense pain in the lower right abdominal area, which is where the appendix is located. I went to the emergency room and had a CT scan done to see if my appendix had burst. It had not burst, and there was no immediate emergency, but the doctors determined that the appendix was inflamed and that to help with the pain, it should come out.

The surgery was intended to be quite routine and straightforward; however, it seldom turns out that way for me! It was performed laparoscopically, meaning they inserted a camera just above the pubic bone and another in the lower left area of the abdomen. The appendix was then extracted through a horizontal incision located just below the belly button. While they were attempting to do my surgery, they found a lot of scar tissue in my abdomen that had developed as a result of my first back surgery. When they did that first surgery, they fused my lower back and had to make incisions through my stomach and my back. The surgery had been done 11 years before the appendectomy, and during that time, the scar tissue had built up enough that it needed to be removed. It also could be the result of some of the pain I had been having, so although it was upsetting to learn that the surgery was more invasive than originally thought, it was also wonderful to think that perhaps there was a potential solution for some of my abdominal pain. (Also, during the surgery, it was discovered that I had a small ovarian cyst, but apparently, it is somewhat common for women to develop them, and then they often disappear and do not need any form of treatment or removal. Since that first cyst was discovered, I have had several more develop and then disappear without needing further treatment.)

Although the surgery was a little more invasive than a normal appendectomy, it generally does not take that long to recover from it. However, I had some complications. First, I had more pain than I originally thought because of the removal of the scar tissue. Since I take narcotics regularly for chronic pain, it is sometimes difficult to determine the dosage needed to treat surgical pain. In addition, chronic pain patients sometimes have increased levels of pain because chronic pain alters nerve pathways and increases and heightens the brain's sensitivity to pain signals. Since the medical community has yet to fully understand the complexities of pain, it can be challenging for me to completely understand it as someone living with chronic pain. The second complication was that I got an infection – the scar that the appendix had been removed from started draining, turned a bright red color, and that area of my abdomen was very rigid and painful.

In the end, the removal of my appendix and the scar tissue that had built up from my first back surgery was a success because it prevented my appendix from bursting, and I will never again have to worry about appendicitis. Additionally, it also helped me with some of the intense pain that would cause me to double over because of the scar tissue that was removed from my abdomen, which was a wonderful, unexpected side effect of the surgery.

Stomach and Colon Cancers:

Stomach and colon cancers are prevalent on the paternal side of my family. My paternal grandpa died of stomach cancer in 1978, so although my mother was pregnant with me at the time, I never got to meet him. In addition, my grandpa had multiple siblings with colon cancer. Also, two of my dad's siblings had colon cancer, so most relatives on that side of the family are acutely aware that they need regular colonoscopies to catch it before it begins or in its earliest stages. Colon cancer can be highly treatable because, unlike any type of childhood cancer, you can have regular colonoscopies to catch colon cancer before it begins or in earlier stages.

I had my first colonoscopy in my early 20s, but I had the next one in my early 30s. Typically, people are advised to start having colonoscopies around age 45, but they may be advised to start even earlier with certain risk factors. The reason I had my first colonoscopy so early was due to the stomach issues I had been having for several years, which I explained in a previous section. That turned out to be a good decision because even in my early 30s, the doctors found and removed four precancerous polyps in my colon. At that age, I had already beaten the number of precancerous polyps, also known as adenomatous colonic polyps, that my dad had. This is a lot to have at my age, and given the prevalence of colon cancer in my family, I have been advised to have a colonoscopy every year to every other year, depending on the number of precancerous polyps that had been found in my most recent colonoscopy. So, for example, when four precancerous polyps were found, I was allowed to have a colonoscopy every other year. There was also a series of years where I had 26 precancerous polyps, then 18 the next year, followed by 20 precancerous polyps. During this time, I had to have a colonoscopy every year.

It is scary that I have had so many precancerous polyps because PREcancerous polyps can result in cancer. Yet, this is also just a beautiful illustration of the importance of having regular colonoscopies. Every precancerous polyp that has been removed from my body gives me one less chance of developing colon cancer.

What made me sick, however, was thinking about drinking the colonoscopy prep on such a regular basis because I did not have fond memories of drinking it. I tried every type of prescription drink for colonoscopies, and I threw up each one of them. Then, I heard from a friend that there was a Miralax prep, but that you needed to ask for it. I was able to switch to this prep instead, and I could finally keep everything down that I was drinking. However, given the fact that I had gastroparesis and a slow-moving digestive system, my doctor had me fast for double the regular amount of time AND start the Miralax prep early so that I could do it twice in a row. It sucks doing the prep early and doubling it, but it is so much better for me than drinking anything that I had in the past.

Gastroparesis, Slow Colonic Inertia:

My GI issues seemed to go in waves, where I would not have any problems for a bit, and then I would start having different symptoms that made normal functioning a bit more challenging. In 2016, I was approaching another colonoscopy, and my GI doctor decided that we should also have an endoscopy at that time. Medicine had evolved, and the once catch-all diagnosis of irritable bowel disease was no longer sufficient. More had been discovered about the entire GI system, but it was also helpful that I had both the endoscopy and colonoscopy scheduled to provide some wonderful diagnostics. Both of those tests were scheduled with the doctor who usually performed my colonoscopies. I like to say that he knows my colon well!

Once the endoscopy and colonoscopy had been completed, my GI doctor came to my room to discuss his findings with me. He informed me that I had a rare condition called gastroparesis. Normally, your stomach muscles contract repeatedly to push food through the digestive tract. With gastroparesis, however, your stomach muscles are slowed down, or they do not work at all, which prevents your stomach from emptying properly and fully. My GI doctor said that it looked like there were some potato skins in there, and I had not eaten potatoes in well over one week!

I was given some materials about gastroparesis, and through these materials, speaking with my doctor, and my own research, I learned that gastroparesis could lead to problems with digestion, resulting in nausea, vomiting, and abdominal pain. Other symptoms included abdominal bloating and pain, acid reflux, and a feeling of fullness after only a few bites of food. Gastroparesis can be very difficult on a person's body, and it can cause severe dehydration, malnutrition, and radical changes in blood sugar levels. Furthermore, undigested food in the abdomen could join together and form a solid mass, which could become life-threatening if it blocked food from moving into the small intestine. All of these symptoms encapsulated what I had been feeling and experiencing with my GI issues, and it was nice to finally have a confirmed diagnosis for what I had been experiencing for many years.

Typically, the cause of gastroparesis is unknown; however, some medications can cause gastroparesis, some can mimic its symptoms, and others can make a diagnosed case worse. There is no known cure for this condition, and the only way to treat it is through changes in medication and diet. Since I could not change my medications, I could only help myself through changes in my diet. These changes involve eating smaller meals more frequently, chewing food thoroughly, and gently exercising after eating, such as taking a walk. Additionally, it is important to eat cooked fruits and vegetables as opposed to eating them raw and avoiding fibrous vegetables.

I have known about the gastroparesis for several years now, and it still is a constant learning curve. I know that I make mistakes with my eating habits daily, and that is likely why I experience abdominal pain, diarrhea, and, at times, constipation. I think that the worst thing that I experience, in addition to the pain, is the bloating and swelling of my stomach. This can be quite dramatic, and it can be so uncomfortable when the bloating and swelling are severe. This is why I try to follow the gastroparesis diet, as well as the other guidelines that were previously discussed. It does make a difference.

In addition, not only do I have gastroparesis, meaning my stomach is slow to digest and empty its contents, but my entire digestive system is slow-moving and slow to digest and empty its contents. Again, gastroparesis is the name for the slow-moving digestion of the stomach. Furthermore, slow transit constipation or slow-colonic inertia are the names given to the slow-moving rate of movement in the large intestine, which can result in constipation, abdominal pain, nausea, decreased appetite, reduced bowel motions, and uncontrollable soiling, which I do not experience, thank the Lord!

There is no name given to the entire digestive system functioning at a slow-moving rate, or a name for the parts that are slow-moving between the stomach and the large intestine. I know that diseases are often named after the doctors who diagnose them, as well as the patients who experience them. To be perfectly honest, I do not want the "honor" of having this medical issue named after me. I would much rather be named after something nice! Yet, I fear that people like me will keep having difficulties with a slow-moving digestive system, and little can be done about it until it is identified and named as a problem.

Hemorrhoids, BAM, and SIBO:

I have also had several hemorrhoid surgeries to help get rid of large, painful hemorrhoids. Luckily, this issue seems to have been resolved, at least for now, after the last surgery in May 2021. This last hemorrhoid surgery gave my family and me way more than what we bargained for. The surgery itself went smoothly, and I woke up without any issues from the anesthetic. To go home, I needed to sit up on the bed and walk around the hospital a little bit. So, I sat up momentarily, just trying to catch my bearings. Then, I was encouraged to stand up and start walking around the hospital. My memories are a bit blurry, however, because I guess as soon as I got to my feet, they slipped right out from under me, and I fainted. Luckily, both my husband and the nurse who was helping us caught me, and I remember coming to, moments later, with the two of them staring at me. I was immediately put back into bed and hooked up to monitors. My blood pressure was extremely low, but my heart rate was very high. Putting all of the "evidence" together, it was determined that I was at the beginning of an adrenal crisis, so I was given additional steroids and needed to spend a night in the hospital so that my levels could improve before I went home. I was able to go home the next day and be reunited with my Siamese cat, who was very happy to welcome me home.

After the adrenal crisis, I was extremely exhausted, which is only natural, but it was so wonderful being home from the hospital. I was doing much better...until the following afternoon when I started bleeding heavily from the surgical site. It was so bad that my husband had to bring me back to the hospital, and I was re-admitted to determine why I was bleeding so that we could stop it. I had some blood work done, and it showed that I was severely anemic from all of the blood loss. It was so bad that I required a blood transfusion! After the transfusion, my blood work slowly started to improve, and we were able to move on to the next task – finding out why I was bleeding. Unfortunately, the only way to see this area of the body was to have a colonoscopy, which meant that I had to stop eating and do the Gatorade prep. My colonoscopy was scheduled early in the morning, but I had a rough night because every time I had to go to the bathroom, I would lose a lot of blood. Eventually, they came to get me for the colonoscopy, and we decided that if the colonoscopy revealed something that needed to be surgically repaired, they would immediately bring me to the operating room without waking me up from the colonoscopy.

Once I woke up, I immediately questioned whether I had to have further surgery or not. The nurses told me that there was an artery that had been bleeding, but that it had almost stopped by the time the colonoscopy took place. They cauterized it so that we were sure that everything had been repaired once and for all. After the colonoscopy, I had to spend another night in the hospital, but after that, I was, once again, able to go home. This time, it was for good! Luckily enough, I have not had any issues with hemorrhoids since this surgery in 2021 that resulted in an adrenal crisis, hemorrhaging and bleeding uncontrollably, and the need for a blood transfusion.

I did, however, still experience some minor bleeding from the site where the large hemorrhoid had been removed, which caused us so much grief with the hemorrhaging and blood transfusion for TWO YEARS after the surgery. I continued to see the surgeon for those two years, and we tried everything to get that area to heal and stop bleeding. However, it never healed on its own, and we had to do some exploratory surgery and biopsies to determine the cause of the bleeding and how to fix it. We determined that the reason why it continued to bleed and would not heal on its own was because I was a tight ass. Seriously! My muscles are incredibly tight in that area, and that tightness kept pulling at the surgical site, causing it to bleed and never heal. To fix this issue, I visited a specialist, and in August 2023, he performed a sphincterotomy, which I am sure sounds glamorous. The surgeon cut one of the muscles in that area, thereby loosening it up so that there would no longer be pulling and bleeding at the surgical site from 2021. The surgery worked perfectly, and I can attest that I am still a tight ass!

Today, I continue to experience both constipation and diarrhea, but more commonly, I have bouts of diarrhea. At times, it almost seemed like I had C. diff again, but instead, I was diagnosed with two other conditions that can cause diarrhea when left untreated, and that made a lot of sense with my other medical conditions. Small intestinal bacterial overgrowth (SIBO) takes place when there is an "overgrowth" of the overall bacteria in the small intestine, especially bacteria that are not typically found in the digestive tract. The reason why this happens is because, for whatever reason, whether it is surgery or disease, the passage of food and waste is slowed down as it moves through the digestive tract, creating a breeding ground for bacteria. Considering that my digestive system is incredibly slow-moving and I have been diagnosed with gastroparesis and slow colonic inertia anyway, it makes sense that SIBO could take place in my body. This condition is difficult to diagnose and treat because the symptoms mimic other GI issues that I have, such as nausea, abdominal pain, bloating, diarrhea, loss of appetite, and malnutrition. Yet, once SIBO has been diagnosed, typically by a breath test, it is treated fairly easily with a course of antibiotics and nutritional support.

Finally, you may be aware that the liver produces bile, which is an acid that aids the body in the digestion of food. Typically, the body releases the perfect amount of bile acid, but sometimes it releases too much, or the body cannot use it properly. In these cases, bile salt malabsorption (BAM) can occur. Diarrhea is often linked to this condition, but it is underrecognized and underdiagnosed. For example, about 1/3 of people diagnosed with irritable bowel disease with diarrhea also have bile acid malabsorption issues. This disease is often overlooked as a cause of diarrhea, and it is generally diagnosed with additional health conditions. Treatment options include medications, dietary changes, and sometimes surgery. Luckily, medication to treat this condition, which occurs occasionally, has worked well for me.

Liver Hemangiomas and Adenomas

When I was younger and in my twenties, I had heavy, painful periods, so I was put on birth control to help with this and to make that time of the month a bit more tolerable. I have also had some pain in the area where my liver is located in the past. As a result of both of these conditions, my doctors did some CT scans to investigate and determine a diagnosis. The tests revealed a liver that was completely spotted like a Dalmatian or looked to be littered with freckles. I also had a liver biopsy, which involved being numbed locally in the abdominal area and having a large needle withdraw a small sample of some of the largest tumors on my liver. It reminded me of an ear-piercing gun that punches a hole in your ear. Instead, this punched a hole through my abdominal wall and into my liver, and it was a little more painful than an ear piercing.

After the testing of the sample was complete, I was diagnosed with having two different types of non-cancerous (benign) masses on my liver. Some of the masses on my liver were called hemangiomas, which are a tangle of blood vessels that are completely benign. The second set of masses that I had were called hepatic adenomas, which are also benign iver tumors. These are a bit more uncommon, and they are often linked to the use of estrogen in birth control. Even though these are benign, hepatic adenomas carry a small but significant risk of bleeding, as well as turning cancerous, so I was carefully monitored during this time. Typically, there are no symptoms except for the spotted liver, but for some reason, I occasionally had minimal pain in the area where my liver was located.

To stop the adenomas and hemangiomas from growing and multiplying, I was taken off birth control pills. I tried a few different forms of birth control, but Nexplanon, which is implanted in my arm and does not consist of the use of estrogen, seems to work best for me. Of course, everyone is different, and it is important to work with your healthcare professionals. As a result of this change, however, the adenomas and hemangiomas disappeared, and my liver is now unspotted. If I became pregnant, however, the natural hormones in my body would increase drastically, and this could cause the hepatic adenomas to grow again. The reason why this is dangerous is that the more the adenomas grow, the greater the possibility that some of those benign liver tumors could become cancerous.

Delayed Development, Infertility, and Childlessness

For many reasons, I have not always felt like a "complete" and "normal" woman. I know that it goes back to not developing until I was much older than my peers because I was several years behind them on the growth charts. My journey with endocrinologists began at a very young age because a common side effect of childhood cancer treatments involved endocrine issues, such as hormone deficiencies and gland malfunctions. Now, many more endocrinological late effects are known, but even when I was a child, doctors knew that my treatments left me with growth and body maturity issues. Every year after my treatments, we would visit the endocrinologist during my annual check-ups, and my height and weight were carefully plotted on a chart and compared with the height and weight of "normal" children. I NEVER fell within the norms of that chart, and after my treatments, my body height and weight were a few years behind my actual age. For example, when I was eight years old, my body height and weight were that of a five or six-year-old.

These factors likely contributed to why I did not have a serious boyfriend until I was a senior in high school. I was behind my friends in development with my body, but also with relationships with the opposite sex. I typically always had a "crush" on a guy, and almost always, the boy was older than I by a year or two. This is likely because although I looked younger than my high school classmates, I was mentally more mature than most of them because of the experiences that I had been through and the exposure to so many adults at a very young age. Yet, guys were not interested in me because, at that age, they are typically looking at the physical characteristics of a woman, and I was several years behind my peers.

By the time I got to college, I was getting attention from men and thoroughly enjoying it, but I think that the majority of my classmates already had these experiences. When I was younger, however, I just wanted to be ordinary, normal, and have the same experiences as everyone else. As I grew older, I did come to appreciate being unique and not being like everyone else, but these feelings took much longer to develop.

Another rite of passage for a girl is the menstrual cycle, but we were not even sure that I would be able to get my period because I had a total of 16 radiation treatments to help shrink the tumor. My parents informed me that the doctors and nurses always covered my uterus with an iron apron for protection from the radiation, but the doctors could not definitively say if there was any long-term damage that could keep me from getting my period. Furthermore, the chemotherapy medications that I was given could also damage my reproductive system and render me infertile. Thus, growing up as a child, we were not even sure that my reproductive system worked properly after the toxicity of chemotherapy and radiation treatments, because testing was not done at that time. The doctors told us that if I got a regular period, it might be an indicator that things were working properly, and I could potentially have children.

My mom, however, got her period when she was 16, so she was a "late bloomer." Thus, perhaps I would be a late bloomer, too, and I would need to wait until I was 16 years old or more to see if I could even get my period. Or, perhaps the reason why I did not have it yet was because the cancer treatments did so much damage that my reproductive organs did not work properly. So, the combination of my mother being a late bloomer, me being several years behind my peers on the growth charts, and possible damage from the chemotherapy and radiation made getting my period at an early age something that would not likely happen. Yet, just like any other child, I desperately wanted to fit in and be like everyone else. I remember being at a sleepover when I was in the 8th grade, and all of the girls were discussing their periods. The talk was about cramps, PMS, and the use of tampons vs. pads, and every single girl in that room was talking like she had her period. I did not want to feel left out or feel like this was another thing that made me different from everyone else, so I joined in sparingly, with what I hoped was a well-placed comment here and there.

Finally, when I was 15, I got my period at school and I was so happy. At that time, my dad was a guidance counselor at my school, so I got to call my mom from his office and tell her the news. As strange as it sounds, we all celebrated because this meant that at least part of my reproductive system was somewhat functional. We had no idea if I was fertile or could get pregnant, but getting my period at least showed that my body had some "normal" functions. To my parents and me, getting my period symbolized that despite my cancer treatments, I could still hit "normal" milestones and experience the same things that my classmates were experiencing. With that mentality, I did not mind the awful cramps and side effects that came with having my period because, in my eyes, each month that I had my period could put me closer to one day carrying a child and becoming a mother.

From the earliest of ages, I always wanted to be a mother. I also tried to mother everything from dolls, stuffed animals, and any type of living animal or pet that I ever had. I grew up pretty fast and was very mature for my age because the first years of my life were spent with adults - parents, doctors, nurses, and other medical professionals. I wanted to take care of all the stuffed animals that I got every time I had a chemotherapy treatment. I still have a soft place for stuffed animals because they have been, and still can be, incredibly comforting, and as a child, I wanted to take care of them and love them.

One stuffed animal that was my favorite and that experienced an awful lot with me was Teddy (I thought that I was incredibly clever naming my stuffed bear Teddy). I received Teddy during one of my baby showers, so he had been with me from the very beginning. He also started going to surgeries with me from a very young age, and the medical professionals would dress him up like he was in surgery, so I had that to look forward to when I woke up in the recovery room. Teddy would also sometimes get a bandage in the same area where I would get a bandage, like he had had the same surgery as I did. As I got older, Teddy would still come to my surgeries, but he would remain under my bed with my belongings rather than clutched in my arms.

Teddy has been to every one of my 52 surgeries. Now, he travels in my backpack with me to the hospital and stays in my backpack. I am a bit old to bring him to the operating room at this point, but I still get incredible comfort knowing he is with me in the hospital. I also would hate to lose Teddy or have him get doused with blood during surgery, so he is protected staying in my backpack in my room or with my loved ones.

Ever since I could remember, I have always wanted to have a daughter. My mom and I have an incredibly close, loving relationship and friendship, and we have always been each other's rock and best friend. I could not have asked for a better role model of a parent, in addition to my dad. From a very early age, I knew that I wanted to have a little girl so that I could strive for a similar relationship and friendship with my daughter. This became one of my top wishes or desires for my future, second only to finding "the one."

I will talk more about "the one," otherwise known as Troy, in the next section of the book, but God truly gave me the best possible partner, and I am so appreciative and grateful for this. Next to my dad, my husband is one of the greatest men that I have had the privilege of knowing and having in my life. Before falling in love with Troy, I had never really considered having a little boy when I was younger. I think that part of that was because I could not imagine who my husband would be, so it was difficult for me to imagine my son, and his looks and mannerisms. However, after I met Troy and we fell in love, I knew that I would also be perfectly happy with, and would love to welcome, a little boy who, in my mind, would look like a miniature Troy. Not only would our son look like Troy, but he would also have a similar personality and mannerisms to his father.

I also had some ideas for names for our potential children, and I would bring these names up whenever Troy and I discussed our potential children. For a little girl, I liked the idea of Charlee Rebecca, after both of my parents. And for our little boy, I loved the name of Toryn Charles. It may seem a bit selfish that both names honored my parents, but I liked this idea because our children would have Troy's family's last name. I was pretty solid on these names, and I was blinded by the excitement of seeing what Troy and I could create and raise together. It may seem silly that I have imagined or fantasized about my family, but I think that it may have been a coping mechanism.

Unfortunately, I have learned with all of my medical experiences that life often does not follow the plans that you make for it, and having children and a small family was just not possible for a multitude of reasons. For me, not being able to have children in any capacity hurts deep within my heart and soul, and this has truly impacted me. As a childhood cancer survivor, I have been through many difficult challenges in my life, and the majority of them have been medically related. Not being able to have a child, however, is by far the most painful condition that I have experienced. Yet, this not only impacts me, but it also impacts my husband, and that may be one of the most heartbreaking aspects. Troy would make the best father, and watching him interact with children is so incredibly natural and sweet. It is also difficult to watch this because I cannot help but imagine how he would be with our children and how much he deserves to be a father.

Even though our marriage continues to strengthen, year after year, our situation has been fraught with heartbreak and difficult decisions, and we have altered the direction of our lives as a married couple. Even in my mid-forties, my head knows that having human children is just not possible, but my heart refuses to completely accept it and give up the dream. Troy has always known that having children with me might be incredibly difficult or impossible, and I think that he always kept this in mind so that it was a little "easier" for him to accept the fact that our family would not include human children.

Most women want children because that is what we are "supposed" to do, and some of us even have these built-in maternal instincts that we need to satisfy by having children. Most of the time, the goal is to get married, buy a house, start a career, and have a family, sometimes in this order and sometimes out of order. Getting married is typically the precursor to getting pregnant. A man and a woman will typically get married and eventually have children, and I was no exception. Troy and I had discussed and decided that, ideally, we wanted two children, a girl and a boy, and that we would first have a biological child, and then we would adopt a baby of the opposite sex to create our family. Before our wedding, we had to go through several sessions of spiritual counseling. One of our sessions included each of us filling out a survey about how we felt about money, religion, working, and, of course, children. Not to brag, but Troy and I had the same answer or expectation for every part of the survey, which was the highest score our Pastor had ever seen, and which seemingly indicated that we were highly compatible with each other.

After getting married, we decided to wait a few years before having children because we wanted to concentrate and focus on each other and cultivating our relationship. That is what my parents did, and we wanted to become a bit more established as a couple before having a baby, as well as save up some money and try to get out of our tiny shoebox apartment because raising a baby would be very difficult in that setting. It would be nice to be able to purchase a house before having a baby, so that is where our thoughts were at the beginning of our relationship. So, this is what we had decided at the time, and we were not really in a hurry because, compared to how my back is now, the pain was a lot less. Additionally, I had a lot fewer medical issues back then, so if my reproductive system worked correctly, I felt like I could physically have a baby at that time.

My family, however, has always had very strong opinions about me getting pregnant, and they are deep-rooted. Remember, I had a chemotherapy medication with a possible side effect being a weakened heart in times of stress. However, my heart has always tested perfectly, so this fear seems to be unfounded.. The fear of becoming pregnant grew to a fever pitch when the movie *Steel Magnolias* came out in 1989 (I was only ten years old!) The movie starred Shirley MacLaine, Sally Fields, and Julia Roberts, and it was both a comedy and a sad tragedy, but the part that affected me, having a baby, centers around Julia Roberts' character, Shelby. Her character had severe diabetes, and in one of the scenes, she had a seizure. The seizure helps illustrate the difficulties that she has with her condition, and her doctor strongly advised against her getting pregnant. Diabetic mothers have increased risks with pregnancy to both the baby and the mother, especially back then. Shelby, however, did get pregnant, and it was a very uneventful pregnancy, with the mother and the baby being just fine throughout the pregnancy, labor, and the first year of the baby's life. However, when the baby was about one year old, the stress of everything took a toll on Shelby's body and worsened her diabetes, resulting in a seizure and death.

Now, we do not even know for sure if having the baby was a contributing factor to her death. In addition, I do not have diabetes, so the medical conditions that we have are completely different. Yet, my family seems to think that I would suffer the same fate as Shelby if I became pregnant and gave birth to a baby. My family has not wanted me to get pregnant ever since because they became scared and convinced that I would die like Julia Roberts' character, Shelby, in *Steel Magnolias*.

After I broke my sacrum in 2005, my chronic pain dramatically worsened, and I was confined to the bed or couch for an entire year while I healed. After that year, I still experienced problems. I tried to go back to work full-time after I recovered, but my body just could not handle it. I did end up working part-time for a telephone company, but my back just continued to worsen, and I had to stop working a couple of years after starting. At this point, I had FINALLY been approved to receive Social

Security Disability Income (SSDI). If things ever started to improve, I could always try working part-time. Yet, I just continued to worsen to the point where I could not sit up for very long without experiencing severe pain and needing to lie down. So, my husband, family, and I decided that it would be best if I stopped working.

So, in addition to fears about how my body would respond to pregnancy, my loved ones were also very concerned about me physically taking care of a baby. I am in pain all of the time, and at that point, I was on quite a bit of pain medication. Neither of these is very conducive to taking care of a baby. Additionally, you need to be alert and awake to take care of a baby, and that need just grows as the child ages. I have problems with that throughout the day because of the severe pain, as well as from the medication that treats the pain. In addition, I cannot lift anything over ten pounds, and once an infant starts gaining weight, that limit is reached FAST. Additionally, lifting and bending to move a baby in and out of a crib, playpen, or changing table can be very painful for someone with a bad back.

Once the baby continues to grow, he or she becomes more active, and there is no way that my cane and I can keep up. Additionally, not being able to sit or stand for very long is just not conducive to taking care of a child, and I had really never considered these things when I thought about having a baby. Truthfully, I had never thought past getting pregnant because that was such a HUGE hurdle and issue to overcome.

This brought on new waves of depression because the dream of having a child just continued to slip away each day, each month, and each year. Various New Year's, birthdays, and anniversaries came and went, and my medical issues and chronic pain just increased with age. I do have a birth control implant in my arm at this point, so we have never actively tried to become pregnant. I have always been very diligent about birth control and being responsible because there are so many medical issues that need to be addressed before we can even try having a baby.

Furthermore, even though I got my period and my reproductive system was working in that way, we did not know if my eggs had been damaged during my cancer treatments. Due to being treated so long ago, I never had any appointments about my fertility, nor were there any discussions about this topic until I initiated them after I was married. I never had any fertility tests. Tests involving fertility can be incredibly expensive, and I am not sure that my insurance would cover it. Early in our marriage, we struggled a bit financially. Depending on insurance and the copay of any testing, it would have been difficult for us to pay for the testing until later in our marriage, when my health insurance was more robust and covered more out-of-pocket expenses.

I had grown to dislike my birthday a bit because, as I got older, the time when I could potentially have a baby was drastically disappearing. I want children more than anything in the world, and getting married and having a family is not only the American dream, but it was also my dream and my husband's dream. However, this dream just slipped away each year due to my possible infertility issues, my aging body, and all of my medical issues and late effects. Despite everything against us, I still wanted to try to have a baby. Even thinking it seemed somewhat delusional, given everything that my body was screaming at me. Despite this, my husband made a deal with me and told me that if my doctors said that I could get pregnant and that the pregnancy would have no long-term effects on me, we could try to have a baby.

My husband is very wise and intelligent, and he knew that most, if not all, of my doctors would NOT give me their blessing to get pregnant. My parents were also on board with this plan, and again, the scenes of Shelby in Steel Magnolias were on their minds. In my head, I pretty much knew that my body would have an extremely difficult time handling a pregnancy. I needed to hear this from a doctor, however, to accept and come to terms with my situation. Yet, if the high-risk OB-GYN said that it would be okay to pursue a pregnancy, then I would go in that direction.

In April 2013, Troy and I went to an appointment with the high-risk OB-GYN. I was not feeling very positive about the appointment, and I was so nervous in the weeks leading up to the appointment, as well as that day. We were led to an examination room that was papered with pregnancy and baby posters and signage. Just seeing these images was heartbreaking, and I know that most of the people who are led into these rooms are pregnant or trying to get pregnant. The posters apply to them, but I could not help but think of the heartbroken people who cannot get pregnant or are having an extremely difficult time getting pregnant, as well as the couples who experienced miscarriages, stillbirths, and infant deaths. It would be incredibly difficult for these people to see pictures of babies. Additionally, my appointment had not even started yet, but Troy and I saw these images of pregnancy and infants, knowing that we would probably be told that we could not have a baby. Perhaps there should be rooms, or at least a room, in this department that are baby-free and pregnancy-free, and then put patients in these rooms accordingly. Whenever I saw those images before this appointment and at subsequent appointments, the posters made me sad, and I felt like they were mocking me or shaming me to feel even worse for not being able to have a child.

The doctor entered our examination room, and just to give you a preview, it was an incredibly short appointment. There was no examination, and very little information was gathered from me because the doctor had read my medical records, which honestly is a feat in itself. The doctor began by saying something like, "98% of women who think they could have a high-risk pregnancy have no reason to worry. Therefore, only 2% of women do need to worry about a high-risk pregnancy, and you," he said, "are in that 2%." The doctor also stated that for me, there would only be about a 2% chance that both the baby and I would survive. He went on to list just some of the top reasons why I should never get pregnant, and honestly, the reasons that he gave us were things that we had not even thought of before the appointment. We thought he would lead with my back being fused, as well as the chronic severe pain. Not only would pregnancy most likely increase my back pain, which I do not even know if I could handle any more pain than I already have, but I would have to quit taking all of my pain medications. I also have weak bones, so the weight of a baby could be too much for my bones to handle. In addition to taking a variety of medications to treat my pain, I also take a slew of medications for other issues, such as depression, kidney disease, asthma, migraines, and a variety of stomach issues. For any pregnancy, we knew that I would have to stop taking most of my prescriptions that I take daily for some serious medical conditions. I would stop taking these medications for the sake of the baby, but my body could suffer from not taking some of my medications.

In addition, we thought that we would also hear about my cancer treatments complicating a pregnancy. As a reminder, I had 16 radiation treatments to my chest, and I had an experimental protocol of chemotherapy medications for two years. It was discovered that one of the chemotherapy drugs that I had can weaken a patient's heart in times of stress. My heart has always tested normally, and I have never had any problems, but giving birth is an incredibly stressful event on a woman's body, and there could be issues with this. We knew that because of my back and the chemotherapy drug, I would never be able to give birth vaginally and that I would need to schedule a C-section.

So, those are the reasons that Troy and I thought would complicate a pregnancy and that the doctor would bring up during this appointment. Yet, as indicated previously, we would hear some additional reasons from the doctor that had not crossed our minds. One of those additional reasons that he mentioned was that my kidney disease would worsen with a pregnancy, and kidney damage is irreversible, so depending on the severity of the kidney disease after the pregnancy, I could face kidney failure and need dialysis or possibly a kidney transplant. The organ transplant list is so long, and the demand is incredibly high, yet the supply of organs is low. Luckily, with a kidney, you can have a living donor because the human body can survive with one working kidney. However, that does not mean that it is easy to find a donor.

The doctor also said that my asthma and restrictive lung disease would severely worsen as the pregnancy progressed. The baby lies below the diaphragm, and the larger the baby grows, the more it pushes up on the diaphragm, and the more I would struggle with breathing. My breathing difficulties are made worse by the curvature of my spine, which remains significant despite the spinal fusion. You might recall that my right lung is nearly half the size of my left lung and functions at only 50% of its capacity. Additionally, my chest wall has caved in on the right side, and that has contributed to some of my right lung restriction. In summary, as a baby grew, I could have more and more trouble breathing from these complicated breathing issues.

The third major reason that the doctor explained why I should not get pregnant was my endocrinology issues, which Troy and I had never even thought about when we discussed the medical issues that may complicate a pregnancy. Taking a thyroid supplement daily does not complicate a pregnancy, but my adrenal insufficiency disease would truly complicate a pregnancy. To treat the adrenal insufficiency disease, I have to take regular doses of prescription oral steroids, which give my body the cortisol levels that it needs to function properly. If I do not get this medication, I could go into an adrenal crisis and then into an adrenal coma, and death. However, taking as much of this medication as is needed to treat my condition may not necessarily be good for the baby. There are very few studies on women with Adrenal insufficiency disease and using oral steroids throughout pregnancy and the effects on a fetus and the baby after it has been born. However, any regular use of medication could affect the baby in some way, and unfortunately for me, taking oral hydrocortisone is necessary.

After the doctor delivered the information and his reasons why I should not have a baby, he then stated that there were many other issues and reasons why I should not become pregnant. He told Troy and me that if I became pregnant, it was highly doubtful that both the baby and I would be healthy and not have any long-term medical effects from the pregnancy. He even stated that there was little chance that both the baby and I would survive. I was somewhat prepared to hear this from the doctor because we had pretty much determined that he would tell us that I should not get pregnant. Yet, it was still incredibly tough to hear, and I tried to keep it together as much as I could while the doctor was there, but I know my eyes were sparkling with tears, which turned into a torrent of tears once we got out of the examination room and into the privacy of our car.

The high-risk OB-GYN doctor ended by saying that under no circumstances should I become pregnant. He then suggested I get my tubes tied and handed me a brochure, which really upset me. Tying my tubes felt so final, and I just couldn't handle that on top of everything else. Even now, I still struggle with the idea. Maybe I'm hoping for some medical miracle, and if my tubes were tied, that hope would be gone. I know it's unrealistic. I simply can't have a baby, but maybe I could still hold onto a sliver of hope. I've always been extremely responsible with birth control and currently have the Nexplanon implant, which lasts three years. Since getting married, I've always used some form of birth control. I even had an IUD before the wedding to be prepared, but during our first year of marriage, it fell out of place and ended up between my uterus and cervix. We were lucky I didn't get pregnant—at least, that's what we said at the time. Looking back, Troy and I had planned to wait a few years before having kids to enjoy time together. But in February 2005, I fell and broke my sacrum, and things have gone downhill since. Before that, the pain I had was nothing compared to now, and I was even working full-time. I also had fewer health problems (some weren't even diagnosed yet), so in hindsight, that may have been the best time for me to get pregnant. But hindsight is 20/20, and there are no do-overs. I've thought about this over and over again, analyzing every angle and possibility. Still, I have my answer from the doctor, and now Troy and I have to move forward, adjusting our expectations and redefining what our future looks like.

Yet, when I was first told by the high-risk OB-GYN that I could NOT have any children, I had an honest conversation with Troy and wanted to give him an "out." We got married thinking that we could have children, but since we were not able to because of my medical conditions, I offered Troy the option of divorcing me and finding a new woman to marry who would be able to give him some children, because that is what he deserved. I know that Troy loves children and wanted to have them, and to be honest, children love and gravitate to him. He is amazing with children and would make the most incredible dad, so I honestly wanted him to consider leaving me. Because Troy is a wonderful person and husband, he assured me that he did not need to have children to be happy and that he would rather be with me. He also pointed out the wedding vow of "for better or for worse, in sickness and in health."

I am incredibly grateful that Troy decided to stay with me, and we reassured ourselves that we would still have an amazing life together and enjoy just being together and focusing on each other, rather than children. We also said that we would be amazing pet parents who would treat our pets like they were our children. We do not want to be seen as weird cat people, so only close people know how crazy we are about our past cats and our current cat, and how important they are to us since we cannot have children.

When someone cannot have a biological child, people try to be helpful and mention that they should just adopt or foster a child instead. To many, this is not a "replacement," and they are offended that adoption is so easily thrown out as a solution to not being able to have a biological child. Women often want the experience of pregnancy and carrying a baby, and knowing that the baby has their DNA, as well as DNA from their husband or boyfriend.

While I respect others' views on adoption, I'm not easily offended by such discussions. Troy and I have always wanted both a biological child and to adopt or foster, especially knowing how many children need loving homes. This was our plan even before learning I couldn't conceive biologically. We hoped for one biological child and then to adopt one of the opposite gender, giving us both a boy and a girl, one biological and one adopted. But as my medical conditions worsened and time passed, adoption and fostering became less realistic. Now in our forties, with my health challenges, I no longer feel capable of caring for a child, which is heartbreaking. Due to the long-term effects of childhood cancer, I live with severe, chronic pain and spend much of my time resting on the couch. Though I try to volunteer from home, most household tasks fall to Troy, who also helps care for me daily. I would never want a child to take on that role. I would want to care for them, let them enjoy childhood without adult responsibilities. I also want to be active in my child's life, playing, attending events, and going on outings. But even simple activities leave me exhausted for days. It wouldn't be fair to a child to have a part-time mom who is largely confined to a couch.

Even though I have many serious reasons not to have a child, and I cognitively have recognized this, I am devastated, and it breaks my heart that I have essentially been forced by childhood cancer to live a life of childlessness, and so has my husband. I do recognize that things are better and easier to handle now, as opposed to directly after that appointment with the high-risk OB-GYN. However, this situation is a grieving process, and sometimes I am okay with everything, while at other times it just hits me.

In addition to wanting to have children since I was a little girl, as well as a desire to have a mother-daughter relationship similar to what I have with my mom, I wanted to see what a baby would look like that was part of me and part of Troy. I also wanted to experience pregnancy. I know that some people have awful experiences with pregnancy and that there are a lot of negative qualities that come with carrying a baby. Yet, I wanted to feel both the good and the bad parts of pregnancy. I especially wanted to know what it felt like to grow a baby and then feel the kick of that baby, from the tiny flutters to the strong kicks of a maturing fetus. I would love to hear the heartbeat and see the baby's first picture from the ultrasound. Way into the future, I would melt for someone to say to me, "I love you, Mommy." It hurts, like a knife to the heart, that I will never get to experience a little one fiercely hugging me and saying those four words, which are the sweetest, most loving words that I know I will never hear, yet I still ache for it. Thinking of never hearing that is probably what hits me the most, because to hear a child say that to you is such a powerful expression of love and affection. Yet, this will never happen for me, and it sucks, and I have cried so much about it. I went through a "Why me?" stage, but in order to get through this and try to prop myself up, I cannot focus on that.

Troy and I have talked about the options that we could pursue to have a biological child, such as in vitro fertilization (IVF). IVF consists of extracting mature eggs and fertilizing them with sperm to create an embryo, all accomplished outside of the body in a laboratory. The embryo or embryos are then implanted into a uterus. This may sound like an easy process, but it is a very difficult, invasive, time-consuming, and expensive endeavor.

In our situation, we could not implant embryos into my uterus, so we would need to use a gestational carrier, or a surrogate. Typically, it would be an incredibly difficult decision to choose someone to carry a baby; however, this decision could be easy for us because Troy's sister, Anna, said that she would be our surrogate. I trust Anna completely, and this would be such an incredible event, but Troy and I just cannot afford this process. Almost none of it is covered by insurance. The complete IVF journey, which includes egg extraction, fertilization of the egg with sperm to create one or more embryos, implantation of the embryos, and the medical expenses associated with such a pregnancy, is simply too overwhelming for us to bear financially.

Stereotypically, our adult lives are mapped out, and people are continually trying to think ahead and ask about the next phase in life. Before college begins, you are asked about your major, but many people end up changing their major, or they end up going through a period of discovery and exploration to decide on their education and future occupation. Once school is wrapping up, people want to know what your job is going to be. When you meet that special someone and are in the dating stage, people wonder when you are getting engaged. But once you get engaged, you are immediately questioned, "When is the wedding?" When you are at your wedding, yes, on your wedding day, people are asking you when you are having children. So, people are continually asking about the next phase in your life, and they follow these stages because they are comfortable and familiar.

Not everyone adheres to this life plan, and there are various reasons for that. You might find it challenging to stick to this roadmap for several reasons. For instance, you may simply choose not to follow it, or you might prefer to approach things in a different order, which can certainly unsettle traditionalists. Alternatively, you might be in a situation like mine where following the plan isn't feasible. This, too, can make others uncomfortable. In these moments, when I can't respond to questions about having children as expected, I often feel like I'm failing in multiple ways. I am unable to give my husband, who would be an incredible dad, the gift of children, nor can I provide both sets of potential grandparents with grandchildren. When Troy and I got married, we anticipated having kids a few years down the line, but due to my medical conditions, I could not fulfill that role as a wife. This leaves me feeling like a failure, and I must confront those feelings. Hearing the question about having children is particularly painful, but I continue to hope that answering it will become easier over time. This situation underscores the fact that when you can't have a child or even try for one, you undergo a process of grief and mourning. While I wouldn't want to equate this with the experiences of women who have faced stillbirths or miscarriages, I sincerely wish for all these situations and the couples involved to be approached with the compassion, care, and kindness they truly deserve.

I am not sure that my heart will ever fully accept that I cannot have a child, whether adopted or biologically. I think part of it is just the way that I was raised and have been taught to think and be hopeful. But every year, shortly after Mother's Day, my birthday arrives on May 24. Another year older means another year without a child, without the hope of a child, and a year closer to the time when I will never be able to have a child because of my age. Please, though, do not think that I am not grateful to be alive because I am so very grateful for that. But each year, my body seems to break down and hurt a little more, and the hope for a child grows more distant.

While Troy and I were coping with our childlessness, I was also worried about our parents missing the opportunity to become grandparents. Troy's mom and dad already had a granddaughter, as Anna's husband, Justin, had a daughter named Libby from a previous relationship. Anna has known Libby since she was one year old, meaning she has almost been a part of Libby's entire life. Anna and Justin also had their first child, Toryann, so now Troy's parents had two granddaughters. My parents, on the other hand, may not be able to experience becoming grandparents, and that makes me feel sad because they would be wonderful grandparents. I do have a brother, but he has always said that he does NOT want to have any children. My parents often hear about their friends' grandchildren. They always deal with it so well. They listen and reassure people that it is okay to talk about grandchildren. I try to follow their example when others talk about their children, but it often comes with twinges of disappointment and pain. I try not to let others see that side of me, but it can still be difficult. Luckily, my family reassures me that they would rather have me in this world than a baby, so it is nice to hear that.

Neurogenic Bladder

When I was a child, I used to wait to go to the bathroom until the last possible minute because I did not want to interrupt playing with my toys. However, my mom used to tell me that I should not do that because I would develop problems when I was older. Unfortunately, she was correct, but the likely cause of my issues stemmed from either primary or secondary cancer late effects.

During high school, my problems with my bladder began. I was able to hold my urine for so long that my bladder became very stretched and distended. I was never able to fully empty my bladder, so it stayed that way. Eventually, there were times when my bladder became so full of urine that I was unable to go to the bathroom and empty it. To help combat this and to slowly shrink my bladder back down to its normal size, I had to learn how to catheterize myself. The plan was to go to the bathroom as much as I could on my own, and then I needed to catheterize myself so that I could get the remaining urine out and slowly start to shrink my bladder back down to its original size.

This plan was okay to follow at home, but I did not want anyone to know what I was doing at school. Luckily, my dad worked at my high school, and he was able to arrange for me to go to the bathroom in the main office. That bathroom would hold my catheter supplies, and there was a door to the office that led directly to the bathroom. Also, that part of the office was shrouded in file cabinets, so I could come and go from the bathroom without encountering office traffic. Honestly, I am not sure if anyone noticed the fact that I went to the bathroom in the main office, but no one ever said anything to me or teased me about doing so, and that was all that mattered to me. I did not need another thing to make me different from my classmates, so catheterizing myself became another medical secret that I kept.

Eventually, about one year after the catheterizing procedure started, my bladder shrank back down to a normal size, and I was able to go to the bathroom without catheterizing myself every time. However, ever since it started in high school, I have always carried around catheterizing supplies because there are times when I am just not able to go to the bathroom. This can happen in my normal life, but it also would occur after I had surgery because it would take a while for my bladder to "wake up" after having anesthetics. It would be so frustrating because whenever I have had surgery, I have had an IV giving me fluids. These fluids circulate through the body, but they also increase how much you need to urinate. My bladder would fill up, and it would be frustrating because I was unable to get my bladder to cooperate and start working. It can be incredibly painful when the bladder fills up when you are staying in the hospital after surgery, and the nurses would need to call the "Cath Team" to come and catheterize you and remove the urine from your body. This would happen quite often because of the IV, and we would need to continually call the Cath Team until my bladder started working again.

Ultimately, I received a diagnosis for my bladder dysfunction, which was identified as a neurogenic bladder. Normally, nerve signals inform the brain and the muscles that regulate the bladder when to contract or relax. However, in a neurogenic bladder, the nerves and muscles do not coordinate effectively, leading to issues with filling or emptying the bladder. In my situation, my bladder struggled to empty, necessitating assistance through catheterization.

Today, my neurogenic bladder has improved drastically, even when I have surgery. Everything started to improve after my last major back surgery in 2014. During that procedure, my entire thoracic and lumbar spine was fused, and an unexpected yet wonderful outcome was the significant improvement of my neurogenic bladder. Since spinal cord and nerve issues can lead to a neurogenic bladder, it's possible that this condition improved when my back was fused and aligned as much as possible. Regardless of the reason, I still carry catheters with me, but I only need to use them a few times each year, which is a remarkable improvement compared to high school and the need to cath multiple times on a daily basis.

Breast Cancer Risk and Reconstruction

Due to the neuroblastoma occurring on the right side of my chest, a significant amount of breast tissue had to be removed to eliminate as much cancer as possible. Initially, it was unclear how much tissue had been taken out and whether I would experience partial growth or none at all on that side. Ultimately, my right breast did not develop, leaving me completely flat, while my left breast grew normally. As a result, I needed to use padding and prosthetics on the right side to achieve balance with the developing breast on the left.

I also did not develop as early as the other girls in my class, which was difficult because guys at that age wanted to look at someone with curves. I also have always looked younger than I was, and I heard it all the time from people, which drove me crazy when I was younger. Now, in my 40s, it is quite nice to hear that I look younger than my age. Yet again, here was something else that made me feel like a freak. I just wanted to have a womanly body that developed symmetrically and at the same rate as my classmates so that I could look comparable to them.

Throughout junior high and most of high school, I just did not appeal to the guys at my school, even though I had some strong crushes. The boys in my grade were very immature, so I tended to like the older boys better, but they were not interested in someone who was developing so late and looked like a child. Furthermore, I guarded my secret that I did not have two regular-sized breasts. But one incident in 6th grade haunts me to this day. One of my male classmates grabbed a large kickball, put it under his shirt on one side, and said, "Hey, everyone. Look. I'm Mariah." At that moment, I could not keep it together, and I ran into the school and into the bathroom to cry. Some friends came in after me and tried to comfort me, but my breast issues were my deepest, darkest secret, and now they had been announced on the playground.

I *never* talked about this, and was dumbfounded that he would even know about my right breast not developing. He mentioned that the mother of one of my male classmates shared this information with her son, claiming that she had learned it from my mother. Immediately, I ran to my mom, and she was just as dumbfounded as I was because she had never really talked to this woman, and supposedly, she had shared my secret with someone she hardly knew. To this day, I still do not know how they found out about this information, but this incident was extremely difficult to get over and even more difficult to forget. Furthermore, it set the stage for some additional bullying in junior high school.

Many of the girls in my class were not very nice to me either, especially when we hit junior high. Part of the problem was that I developed so much later than they did. Once we got to junior high, everyone started wearing bras. So, even though it was completely unnecessary, I also started wearing a bra in junior high so that I could be just like my classmates. One day, we changed for gym class, and I realized that I forgot to put my bra on that morning. It was such a new thing to me to wear a bra, and as I said, it was completely unnecessary, so I did not have this built into my morning routine yet. The girls in my class noticed, and even though some of these girls used to be some of my best friends in elementary school, things changed when I got to junior high. I guess the girls discussed the fact that I was not wearing a bra that day because when we were running laps, my former friends and other female classmates would run by me, say hi, and then slap me on the back where a bra should have been to embarrass me because I did not have a bra on that day. The tears flowed that night, but I never forgot to wear my bra again.

Once I was old enough, I elected to go ahead with reconstructive surgery to make my right breast the actual size it should have been. All of this was covered by insurance because it was the result of having had cancer in the chest or thoracic cavity. However, the outcome has been very disappointing because, in the beginning, the scarred, radiated tissue kept squeezing the implant. Additionally, even though the implant was stitched into a pocket, it continued to migrate toward my armpit. Due to both of these issues, as well as having a real breast that is not as "perky" as my implant, I had to have a series of several breast reconstructive surgeries. One surgeon even estimated that I would need this surgery every two to three years. My left breast, which has a small implant for symmetry's sake, needed a regular breast lift to make it more symmetrical with the right side. It has taken many years to get to where I am today, and I am quite fortunate that any work could be done on the right side because of the radiation scar tissue that is located there. Yet, I am unhappy with the overall results because I still do not have symmetry, and my body bears quite a few scars from these surgeries.

Men seem to love women's breasts, and mine are just not quite right, which makes me feel like less of a woman. There are times when I even dislike letting my husband see me with the lights on because of my breasts. My husband is the most wonderful man, though, and my feelings are not a reflection of how he feels. He loves me just the way that I am, and I am so lucky to have found him. Even with his love, part of me continues to pursue symmetrical breasts because, again, this makes me feel like a freak and less of a woman.

Visually, there is quite a difference between the two breasts, enough to require some extra padding on the right side to attempt to even things out. During my childhood, I wanted and longed to have a womanly body that developed at the same rate as my classmates, and that would give me the perfect breasts. As an adult, however, I know that perfect symmetry does not exist, especially with women's breasts. Women often have different-sized breasts, and by attaching more logical thinking to this matter and removing the emotion, my goal is now to just have breasts that look as symmetrical as possible under a shirt, with a bra, and without any extra padding.

It was after one of these reconstructive surgeries that we heard that my chest wall had "caved in" on the right side. I remember waking up from anesthetic after surgery, and being terrified when the surgeon told my family and me this news. He had informed us that my "chest wall was caving in," and I remember the fear that I felt while lying in bed and being in such a vulnerable position. My mind was foggy because I was just waking up, and I believe that I asked my parents a few times about the news that we had heard because I could not figure out if it was real or not. When it was confirmed as being real, I felt so much fear and anxiety, and I wondered if my chest would just fall on top of my lungs and heart, making me unable to breathe, and my heart would stop beating.

When I had a CT scan of the thoracic area of my body, it showed that the right side of my chest wall had likely caved into its current position directly after my cancer treatments. The spectacular news is that it is unlikely to cave in any further. There is always the possibility, but as I get older and the chest wall remains at the same angle, it is unlikely that this will happen. We are working with a surgeon to monitor this situation, and when previous X-rays were compared to more recent ones, my chest wall remained stable.

My asthma may be attributed to the deformities within my chest wall, but this is being treated with a preventive prescription, as well as an inhaler, and it is typically only a problem during physical activity, extreme stress, or illness. There is a possibility that the chest wall could aggravate my asthma, but doing something about it could potentially aggravate the asthma even further. Therefore, we are working toward alleviating some of the pressure on the right side of my chest, which my doctor is confident will halt it from caving in even more. We did speak briefly about the possibility of "propping up" the chest wall to restore it to the same position as the left side. However, this would involve introducing foreign material into the chest cavity, which means that there would be a high probability of the introduction of a life-threatening infection in the cardiothoracic cavity. Therefore, we decided to go with a less invasive procedure that should eliminate any additional caving in of my chest wall.

At this point, we are also dealing with my chest wall and how it is affecting the placement of my implants. Before my mastectomies, I needed reconstructive surgery on my chest every few years because the right implant kept shifting up and toward my armpit. It would not even be close to symmetrical, and it would be located so far under my armpit that I could not even put my arm down fully because the implant would be in the way. The implant had been stitched into place, and that helped keep it in place for a bit. Yet, like something at the top of the hill, the implant keeps shifting because of the positioning of the chest wall. There is a very complicated, risky surgery that could maybe keep the implant in place more permanently. However, nothing is certain, and I believe that the risks far outweigh the benefits, and the procedure is not even guaranteed to work. A possible and permanent solution would be to have nothing in my chest, but I would feel incomplete as a woman and completely self-conscious.

I also remember waking up from another reconstructive surgery and hearing bad news again. After that surgery, I was told in the recovery room that the doctor had cut my lung by accident, and I had to have a chest tube to reinflate the collapsed lung. This news also seemed crazy and unbelievable to me at that time, as well. Receiving difficult news after two of my reconstructive surgeries has made me feel just a little fearful about what news will be told to me once I wake up from anesthesia.

In addition to the various surgeries that I have had to address breast symmetry, monitoring for breast cancer has also become a concern. Since my tumor was attached to my heart and spine, I had radiation to my chest, and that increases my risk for breast cancer. I also had doxorubicin, which, as you have read, is an anthracycline, and it can also cause breast cancer in childhood cancer survivors. If I ever were to get the disease, it would need to be caught early for me to have a chance at survival. Since my radiation treatments were to the chest for my neuroblastoma treatments, I cannot have any radiation for breast cancer because you cannot have radiation to the same area of your body. So, I started breast cancer screening at the age of 28 with mammograms and an MRI. The reason why an MRI was needed was that this screening method would give me a better chance at early detection than a mammogram alone. For my first MRI, my medical insurance did not appreciate this "invasive" technique, and they said that they were not going to pay any of the $4,000 bill. After a letter from my doctor, however, they finally agreed to pay the portion that they were supposed to, and they have continued to pay for the MRI ever since that initial one.

Although I was not expecting to have any problems with my mammogram or MRI, the doctors saw and felt something that seemed suspect in my first round of tests, resulting in a breast biopsy. It was so scary to once again face a possible cancer scare, and my poor parents had to deal with it as well. Since I did not have the comprehension of a "cancer scare" during part of my childhood, I was less of a veteran at it than my parents, but due to personal experience later in life, I have learned that it does not get any less scary or easier to deal with. My husband, however, has that wonderful attitude of taking things as they come and not worrying about things until you have to. Therefore, he was concerned about the "spot," but he was not going to "freak out" until he knew for sure it was cancer. So, my mom came with me to the biopsy appointment, which was later in the day. I had a few other appointments at the Mayo Clinic that day, so to help occupy our minds, we went shopping and tried to have a fun day together. The biopsy itself was not very painful or invasive, and the area where the tissue was taken was marked with a tiny angel wing so that we knew that area had been tested in the future.

The difficult part of the whole ordeal was the waiting and trying to remain patient until the results were in. Thankfully, we learned fairly quickly that the lump was scar tissue and that there was nothing to worry about. I have had many screenings since that time, and every time there has been no evidence of breast cancer.

Since the biopsy, I started working with my local high-risk breast cancer clinic. They determined that due to the radiation to my chest, I had a 5-20% higher risk of getting breast cancer, but I was only informed that this applied to the left breast. You will likely remember that my tumor was on my right side, so all of the radiation was aimed at that area. Yet at first, we were essentially told that there was not enough breast tissue on the right side for us to worry about a mastectomy on that side. Furthermore, it was difficult to determine an exact risk percentage because although I did have radiation to the chest, it was when I was only one year old. Due to the increased chance of contracting breast cancer, screenings are extremely important. Therefore, the medical professional that I worked with at this clinic determined that every six months, I would get a mammogram, and then 6 months after that, I would alternate and get an MRI, and so on. Additionally, I would see my medical professional for an appointment and a manual breast examination every 6 months after both the mammogram and the MRI.

This went on for years until we were told that my risk assessment for contracting breast cancer on the left side was higher than what was originally assessed. The reason why is that we were told at that time that there was not enough remaining breast tissue on the right side of my body to even worry about contracting breast cancer on that side. (That assessment would later prove to be wrong, as you will read shortly.) Yet, we needed to worry about my left breast because of the scatter radiation that I had received. So, because of the risk and the fact that I could not have radiation to the chest again, I chose to get a prophylactic, or preventive, mastectomy of the left breast in January 2017. Since that was the side of my body that was not directly radiated, and it was also the side that had the lesser number of reconstructive surgeries, that surgery was fairly simple and uncomplicated. I was just sore for a bit of time, but to be comfortable, I put a small pillow under my left arm. Luckily for me, since the left side had much less scar tissue and radiated tissue than the right side, the surgeon was able to put in an implant immediately. Once the surgery was complete, things already looked more symmetrical on the right side, and I was thrilled with the result.

As things evolved and more information became known about childhood cancer survivorship and late effects related to breast cancer, Troy and I returned to Mayo Clinic in December 2017 to see Dr. Mutter, a radiation oncologist who would be able to tell me if I needed to have a prophylactic mastectomy on the right side of my chest. Because I had radiation to the right side of my chest, and since I had an anthracycline chemotherapy medication, we had already discussed the fact that breast cancer was a high risk for me. Dr. Mutter estimated that I had about a 50-85% chance of developing breast cancer, given the age at which I was diagnosed with neuroblastoma, as well as the treatments that I received. This estimated annual risk of 50-85% was similar to a patient with either the BRCA 1 or BRCA 2 gene mutation. Furthermore, I was once again reminded that I could not have additional radiation to my chest because I already had chest radiation when I was treated for neuroblastoma. Dr. Mutter let us know that I should consider having a mastectomy of the right breast because, even though it did not look or feel like it, there was a lot of remaining breast tissue on that side. Furthermore, he thought that this could also help me gain even more symmetry, which is something I feel like I have been chasing for the majority of my life. The best reason for having the additional mastectomy of the right breast is that it would drastically reduce my chances of getting breast cancer.

Therefore, in June 2018, I had another mastectomy, but this time it was on the right breast. The surgery was very challenging because this was the side that consisted of a great deal of radiated and scarred tissue. The surgeon had informed us that it was possible that we may not even be able to do any reconstructive work on the right side, given that the blood supply would be challenged because of all of the previous surgeries. The surgeon also said that he would need to remove my nipple because of the blood supply issue and because, in one of my previous reconstructive surgeries, the nipple had already been removed and resewn in the center of the newly reconstructed breast. That could not happen again because it was a miracle that it happened the first time. I wish that someone had told me that I was going to need a double mastectomy when I was younger and undergoing reconstructive breast surgeries at that time. Today, it seems so obvious because we know that breast cancer is a secondary cancer when children have had radiation to the chest, as well as an anthracycline chemotherapy treatment. Yet, back then, it was either not known or not communicated to us. Honestly, I did not feel great about losing the nipple on the right side of my body and not the other, which did not speak well for symmetry in my book, but it was necessary, and I had to remind myself that I was doing this to avoid breast cancer. Plus, I was told that I could get a tattoo of a nipple, which would be an extremely realistic depiction. I could not imagine how that would look, especially in the absence of a regular nipple, but I agreed that it was okay to remove it and to have the tattoo after the surgery and the initial healing process.

After a challenging surgery, the majority of the tissue was removed from the right breast, and my right nipple was removed completely. The surgeon was able to insert an expander inside the chest wall so that they could slowly stretch the skin over several months and eventually have enough room to put in an implant and complete the reconstructive surgery on the right side of my chest.

I knew that I would not need to mourn losing my breasts throughout this process because I had felt like I had already done so in junior high and high school. During those periods in my life, my right breast did not develop, while my left one continued to grow. Thus, I needed various reconstructive surgeries after I finished maturing, and despite all of the struggles and multiple surgical attempts, I could never achieve anything close to symmetry because of the scarred, radiated tissue on the right side of my chest. So, I knew that I would be okay with that aspect of the surgery. I was not prepared, however, to have the expander start at the very beginning of the process. After the mastectomy of the right breast, it was extremely difficult to look in the mirror and see a normal breast on the left side and a completely flat, bare space where the right breast should be located. I had implants for so long that I just did not remember, nor did I want to remember, how my chest looked before I got any of my reconstructive surgeries. I was also transported back to junior high and high school, and those feelings of shame and the need to hide this "secret" from everyone. I missed my previous breasts because even if they were not symmetrical, at least I had something on the right side of my chest.

I also had to return to wearing a special bra with a pocket, where I could add something to the pocket to help obtain symmetry. This time, however, it was a bit difficult because, for the first 1 ½ months, I had special tubes on the right side of my chest that helped remove extra fluid from the chest. At first, we discovered that shoulder pads, or better yet, the bra pads that came in swimsuits and workout clothes, were ideal because we could slowly build up that side of the body to make it symmetrical with my left breast. I was also gifted a pair of "Knitted Knockers," which are special breast prostheses that are handmade for women who have had a lumpectomy and/or mastectomy (by the way, the name, "Knitted Knockers," makes me giggle every time I think of it!) Women from around the country will make them for patients like me, and this was just what I needed to make my breasts look symmetrical. As we filled the expander and the breast got larger, I was able to use the Knitted Knockers, as well as one or more bra inserts from swimsuits or sports bras.

Very slowly, and every few weeks or so, we would go to the Mayo Clinic and get my expander filled up with saline. Immediately, I wanted to just fill it up completely so that we could get an implant in there; however, it did not work like that. Patience was required as we slowly filled up the expander because we needed to stretch the tissue that was remaining on the right side of the body. This was especially important because my skin and tissue on that side are extremely paper-thin, so we needed to move like molasses, which, if you are not familiar, moves very slowly and deliberately.

From after my surgery in June 2018 to December 2018, we slowly filled the expander and stretched the skin. In December 2018, I had reconstructive surgery on the right breast, which was described to me as difficult and precarious. The expander was removed, and an implant was inserted that provided the best symmetry with the left side. This implant always had to be quite a large size to accommodate for the chest wall caving in, and this time was no exception. In other words, the implant looked rather large outside of my body, but when it was placed in the desired area, much of the implant was swallowed up by the effects of the chest wall caving in. In addition to a large implant, the surgeon also did some fat grafting to help provide better symmetry with the left side. Further, the surgeon performed a capsulorrhaphy, which involved repairing a tear on the right side that had occurred from previous surgeries. Repairing this tear would also keep the implant from moving around and sliding up or toward my armpit.

Several months after the surgery referenced above, I was able to fully complete the reconstruction of my right breast. I returned to the Mayo

Clinic and the breast cancer floor, and the Physician's Assistant who had helped me all along with my right side mastectomy, and who also filled up the expander every few weeks, just so happened to be the tattoo artist that I could work with to get my nipple tattoo. I was so fortunate to have her on my team because I was extremely comfortable with her, and I trusted her implicitly.

I was informed that I was quite fortunate to undergo this surgery and that it was successful. Furthermore, I was THRILLED with the outcome of the tattoo. It is incredibly realistic! While I understand that perfect symmetry wasn't achievable, this was the best possible result considering my circumstances and the radiation I had on the right side of my chest. For about four years, I felt very content with the results, which is the longest period that I had experienced satisfaction with the symmetry of my breasts after the surgery.

Severe Scoliosis, Fusion, and Chronic Pain

During my cancer treatment, I underwent intense radiation therapy targeted at the tumor that developed and grew OUT of my spine. This radiation resulted in the loss of some of the spongy material located between my vertebrae, known as intervertebral discs. Consequently, we were aware in advance that these radiation treatments would lead to scoliosis in both my thoracic and lumbar spine, a condition referred to as thoracolumbar scoliosis. Scoliosis, which we will examine further, is a curvature of the spine that typically increases during the growth spurt. My doctors and surgeons also suspected that I may have some kyphosis, which is a pronounced rounding of the upper back, also called hunchback. Specifically, it was the collective doctors' and surgeons' opinions that the dosage of radiation that was prescribed would not compromise the spinal cord, but it would result in a reduction in measured sitting height as I reached maturity. However, during my cancer treatments from ages one to three, my doctors and surgeons were unable to predict the severity of my scoliosis. They also could not anticipate that many of the medical issues I would face throughout my life would arise from this condition and the associated pain.

To better understand scoliosis, we must first examine the spine. The spine is generally divided into three parts: the cervical spine, which includes seven vertebrae at the top of the spine, or the neck region; the thoracic spine, made up of twelve vertebrae in the mid-back region; and the lumbar spine, consisting of five lower vertebrae connected to the sacrum or tailbone. In my case, scoliosis affected most of my spine, particularly the thoracic (mid-back) and lumbar (lower back) vertebrae. The radiation treatments were specifically aimed at my thoracic spine, but the resulting curvature impacted the entire spine, including the lower lumbar region. Some of my doctors speculated that I might have had some form of scoliosis, regardless of whether I received radiation to the spine, which could explain the severity of my condition throughout both the thoracic and lumbar sections. Fortunately, my neck, or cervical spine, was only minimally impacted.

Typically, the cause of scoliosis is unknown or idiopathic, and treatment of scoliosis depends on the cause and severity of the curve. Scoliosis is quite common, and many people are diagnosed with it, but most cases are very mild; there are no symptoms, and no treatment is necessary. For me, we knew that the curve originated from the radiation to the tumor growing out of several levels of my thoracic spine. I had a severe case of scoliosis, which can cause chronic back pain, shortness of breath, and deformities. These cases typically need to be treated with surgery.

The signs and symptoms of scoliosis, which are usually first noticed in children around eight years of age, include uneven shoulders, prominent shoulder blades, uneven waist, elevated hips, and leaning to one side.

Doctors categorize scoliosis based on several factors related to the curve. A scoliosis curve may appear as a C or S-shape and may occur in the upper (thoracic) or lower (lumbar) spine, or between the two areas (thoracolumbar). The doctors may also categorize the curve by the direction, angle, or cause of scoliosis. The cause for approximately 80% of scoliosis cases is unknown, but researchers do know that it can have a hereditary component. Risk factors have also been identified, and it was determined that females are more likely than males to get scoliosis. Early detection of scoliosis is also important because the curve has the potential to cause serious health problems, such as severe back pain, difficulty breathing, physical deformities, and injury to the lungs and heart. Therefore, doctors regularly use physical examinations and X-rays to screen and diagnose scoliosis.

The treatment of scoliosis is essential for severe curvature of the spine and may include the use of an orthopedic brace and/or surgical intervention. Braces are typically recommended for curves measuring between 25 to 40 degrees; however, they are not designed to cure or improve the curvature, but they prevent it from worsening. Consequently, bracing is only a viable option during the years of active growth. Physicians may utilize either the full-torso Milwaukee brace or the more discreet thoracolumbosacral orthosis (TLSO). I had the unique experience of wearing both types of braces.

The other alternative, which is generally utilized for curves greater than 40 or 50 degrees, is surgery, which will improve the curve and function of the back. Generally, doctors perform a spinal fusion surgery using instrumentation, which involves placing pieces of bone between vertebrae and holding them in place with metal rods, hooks, screws, and wires. Spinal fusion may also involve opening the chest cavity and fusing from the front of the spine, rather than the back of the spine.

Due to radiation, the intervertebral discs disintegrated at various levels of my thoracic spine, and although doctors informed my parents that I could develop scoliosis, they were unable to predict the severity of the spinal curvature. Additionally, as I grew, the radiation caused my torso to be shorter because of the curvature, so my overall height decreased. Overall, I only grew to be around 5'2", and that was after I gained a little bit of height from multiple fusion surgeries to lessen the severity of my scoliosis curve and straighten my spine as much as possible. Thus, I fought hard to get to this height. I sometimes wonder how tall I could have been without the radiation, or what my height could have been if it were possible to straighten my back completely. Yet, these scenarios just are not possible, so it is not worth it to dwell on something that cannot be changed. Overall, I strive to be happy and positive with the height that I am. And, at least, I reached a height of over five feet.

Throughout my childhood, the curvature of my spine was monitored carefully, and it gradually increased as I grew. We discussed the options with my doctors, and we learned that surgery would probably be the likely outcome in the long run. Yet, spinal fusion surgery is a very serious, invasive, and restrictive procedure, so my doctor wanted to treat my scoliosis very conservatively and save surgery as the last possible option. Since there was a possibility that my spinal curve could be halted or slowed by wearing a back brace, it was determined that this would be the next course of action. To halt or limit the drastically growing curve, I was told that I needed to start wearing a Milwaukee brace. The brace was specially made in an orthotic/prosthetic shop at the Mayo Clinic to fit my body, and I officially received my first back brace on the very first day of 8th grade, so I had to miss that day at school.

To say that junior high was a difficult time for me is an ultimate understatement. Even without a back brace, I felt like a freak and an outsider during junior high, like so many others before and after me. That time was already challenging as students from Galesville, Ettrick, and Trempealeau all merged into one school district for junior high and high school, after attending separate elementary schools. On top of navigating that transition, I lost all of my close friends from elementary school for reasons I didn't understand, which only added to the sense of isolation. They became "too cool" to hang out with me anymore, and since I was so painfully shy because of my insecurities with my medical issues and in general, I had periods throughout junior high when I felt like I had no friends and no one to depend on. There were also many times when I sat alone during lunch. During junior high, my psychosocial issues, including obsessive-compulsive disorder, depression, and anxiety, came to a head, and I thought of suicide on more than one occasion. Again, the back brace was just another thing that made me different.

Furthermore, I was even bullied by both teachers and classmates during lunch. One time, I was trying to get my lunch, and someone slapped my tray out of my hands, sending my food flying all over the cafeteria, leaving a mess on the floor. It seemed like one of the male teachers decided to amuse himself, and although the mess was not my fault, he forced me to grab a huge janitorial mop and clean up the mess that I had made. As you have read, I was a very small child, and the fact that I was also several years behind on the growth chart did not help. The mop was for a large man, and I just could not handle it. I tried with all of my strength to clean up the mess my tray had made, but I was unable to wield the mop. Furthermore, the difficult task was made even more difficult because the teacher and many of my classmates sat there watching me try to handle the mop, pointing and laughing. I felt my cheeks start burning and tears welling up in my eyes, but I pressed on. Eventually, a student came up to me and asked if he could help, and I gratefully accepted his help.

In junior high, appearances are very important, and name-brand clothes were a must to be "cool" and accepted. Now, as an adult, this is so superficial and vapid, but as a pre-teenaged girl struggling to gain acceptance among classmates and friends that I had had throughout my life, this was everything. A bulky back brace was NOT conducive to trendy, name-brand clothing, and I was not able to wear the current trends that my classmates donned. I was very nervous and self-conscious about people seeing the back brace, so I only wore things that covered it. This consisted of turtlenecks and dickeys, which are fake turtlenecks that look similar to a large bib. To this day, I will NOT wear a turtleneck or anything remotely similar to one because it reminds me of my back brace and trying in vain to cover it up. Thus, I was not able to wear any of the cool, trendy clothes, and the clothes that I did wear to attempt to hide the bulky back brace were nice, but they were made fun of and not considered to be cool or trendy. I felt like a freak wearing the clothes that I needed to wear, and people stared at me wherever I went because, despite my best efforts to camouflage the brace, it was there on display at all times.

My doctor did allow me to remove my brace for one glorious hour every day, as well as for P.E. class, much to my dismay. I had been hoping to get out of P.E. class, which is almost every student's nightmare, especially in junior high. I am not athletic at all, however, and I was terrified to take showers because of my physical deformities, so I had hoped that I could get out of P.E. class and let my brace provide one bright side to my life. My doctor, however, wanted me to get a little movement and exercise for the muscles that were held in place by the brace. Unfortunately, I could not remove my brace myself, so my parents talked with my P.E. teacher, and we had a group meeting to show her how to remove my brace, as well as how to put it back on. So, I was mortified because this was something else that differentiated me from my classmates. Are you sensing a theme?

Yet, my P.E. teacher in junior high didn't always follow the instructions to remove my brace during class, and that led to a very frightening incident. We were doing a bicycle riding course because there were and still are some beautiful bicycle trails that bordered the Mississippi River. For some reason, my teacher decided that I didn't need to remove my brace since biking didn't involve twisting. However, balance is critical when riding a bike, and delicate balancing adjustments are nearly impossible in a back brace. I was nervous but tried to participate anyway. Because P.E. classes were only 55 minutes, everything was rushed, from changing clothes, grabbing our bicycles, riding to the trails, and proceeding down the trails as much as possible. I struggled to get on the bike and was urged to hurry. As soon as I began pedaling, I lost my balance and fell, crashing into multiple bikes and riders. It was a large accident, but thankfully, I was the only one injured.

One former friend was angry that her bike had tipped over, but a few classmates were concerned about me. The teacher, however, told everyone to head to the trail and said I could take myself to the nurse's office. One classmate offered to stay and help, but the teacher refused, saying I had already disrupted the class enough. I had hurt my ankle, wrist, and bumped my head. While the injuries weren't serious, I was emotionally shaken. I couldn't believe my teacher, who helped remove and reapply my brace regularly, was so cold and dismissive. I could have had a concussion or a broken bone, yet she left me to manage alone. After the ride, she apologized when she found me in the nurse's office. But her apology couldn't undo how I felt or erase the fact that she had blamed me in front of the entire class.

There was one classmate who continually teased and made fun of me, and for some reason, we always seemed to end up standing in the lunch line next to each other. One day, I just became sick of his teasing and thought about how I could get back at him. There was nothing that I could say that would affect him, so I thought of a physical way to get back at him. My back brace is very hard, and it really could injure someone if they ever were cruel enough to punch me in the stomach. I knew that this guy was cruel enough to do that, so I began to work on putting my plan into action. He was horrible enough to take the bait and punch me, a girl who was at least half his size with multiple medical issues, in the stomach. The expression on his face after he punched me and discovered that my back brace was much tougher than he anticipated was priceless. I think that he almost broke his hand. He did not, but I think that his hand was pretty sore for a while. After all the teasing and the fact that he was cruel enough to punch a tiny, medically challenged girl in the stomach, I got such satisfaction from his injury. When the principal questioned me about the incident, I swear that I could almost see a smile flicker on his face when I explained my side of the story. And just in case you were wondering, I did not get in trouble for the incident either!

The brace was also quite restrictive for me to move around. I was not able to bend, twist, or move when it was on because it did its job by holding my spine in place. Due to this lack of movement, I did occasionally fall over or stumble, and when that happened, I was virtually like a turtle, helplessly lying on top of its shell. Some students recognized this, and there were a few times that I was thrown into the large garbage cans at school. I was unable to get out of the garbage cans on my own because I could not move. I always seemed to be thrown into the garbage cans during the few minutes in between classes, when my other classmates would be walking the halls and going to their lockers to get the materials for their next classes. So, many students would walk by or stand around the garbage cans and stare and laugh at me as I struggled in vain to get out. The only way that I was able to get out of the garbage can was if someone helped me, and by the time that happened, many students had already seen me and laughed at me in this predicament, and I was already in tears. Luckily, the person who always threw me into the garbage can was also the one who would eventually help me get out of it!

As you have read, I am a student who is interested in academics and music. This is because I am not an athlete by any stretch of the imagination, and I am fully aware of that fact. However, I think that my parents wanted me to have the team-building experience of being in athletics, so I started taking golf lessons. Right away, I stood out a bit because I was a left-handed golfer. Additionally, despite taking golf lessons and practicing with some of my teammates on the weekends, I was a horrible golfer. However, my doctor told me that I could remove my back brace whenever I went golfing. I am a rule follower, so this suited me well. Plus, there was no way that I could golf with the brace on because it was too restrictive, and it did not let me bend and flex throughout the entirety of a golf swing. I liked all of the girls on the golf team, so I continued to play golf through freshman year and part of my sophomore year. I am not sure I ever finished better than second-to-last place, but I continued to try until I could no longer do so.

During my sophomore year of high school, I had a horrific injury that ended my golf career. Because I was in a back brace for 23 hours each day, my back muscles were only used or engaged for 1 hour every day. When I was allowed to take the brace off to play golf, I could use those muscles for a little longer each day, but they certainly were not conditioned for that. The result was that I tore and sprained muscles throughout my back during one of our golf meets that was located almost the furthest distance away from our high school. It was an incredibly painful injury throughout my back, and although my parents offered to come get me, it would almost take them too long to get there, so I chose to stay with my team. However, that also meant that I had to ride back home on a bumpy bus for several hours, and I could feel

EVERY. PAINFUL. BUMP.

My doctors determined the diagnosis, and after I healed from this agonizing injury, they decided that I should no longer play golf because there was no way that I could condition the muscles to work for golf but then go back to doing nothing for 23 hours out of the day, minus the time that I was out of the brace for golf practice and meets. They also could not guarantee that an injury like this would not happen in the future, and given how painful it was, I certainly was in agreement with my doctors and retired as a golfer.

Despite wearing the back brace for well over four years, it seemed like the back fusion surgeries were inevitable because I continued to grow crooked and experience back sprains and muscle tears, chronic pain, numbness, and various neural problems. Originally, I had two fusion surgeries. The first was to fuse three levels of my lumbar spine and sacrum using heavy pedicle screws. The second fusion surgery was to fuse levels two through 12 of my thoracic spine using Harrington rods, which left me with the majority of my back fused. However, in 2014, I had to have my entire spine operated on again and re-fused from the top of my thoracic spine down to my sacrum. Additionally, due to severe pain and significant protrusion from my spine, I have had multiple surgeries to remove instrumentation that was put into my back during one of the initial fusion surgeries. Overall, I have had just shy of 10 spinal surgeries, including three significant fusion surgeries. After several very long, brutal surgeries lasting around 10 hours, my back consists of pedicle screws, nuts, bolts, and washers, as well as titanium rods that are fusing everything but my neck. On an X-ray, my back looks like it is housing a small hardware store. Although the scoliosis is stable, my spine still has a significant curvature that will never be fully straightened. Additionally, my doctors informed me of the devastating news that due to the deformities in my back from the cancer treatments, and the severity of my scoliosis, I will always have significant chronic pain that will continue to worsen each year.

Before my first back surgery, which would fuse my lower lumbar spine to my sacrum, I had to wear a body cast for 10 days to simulate the effects of the spinal fusion. The body cast would hold me in a position that was similar to what the fusion would accomplish, and if the pain lessened during that time, there was a greater chance that the fusion would ease my pain. I could not bend at all at the waist, so I had a special wheelchair that allowed me to lie down but still be propped up so that I could attend class. My mom and I affectionately remember that wheelchair because it was made of wood and metal and was extremely heavy. She and I were alone at the Mayo Clinic, and she had to get the wheelchair into the back of our car by herself, which was an almost impossible feat for a single person to do. I was utterly unable to assist as I was confined inside the body cast. After struggling to maneuver the wheelchair into the car on her own with no success, my mom resolved to ask the next man who exited the elevator and entered the parking ramp for help. The next man that entered, however, had a broken arm in a cast and a sling. After laughing at the irony of this, my mom, who is a VERY determined person, took this as a "sign" and decided to try once again to get the wheelchair into our car. She succeeded, which was nothing short of a miracle. Then, we could laugh at the ridiculousness of it all.

The week that I had the body cast was a crazy, exhausting week. First, the only place that I could sleep was on the floor in our living room. I could not get comfortable on my bed in the body cast, and the floor provided me with a bit more comfort. I could not, however, get up off the floor without some major assistance from my parents or my brother. Furthermore, it was my senior year of high school, and I had a full class load plus a ton of music obligations (playing the oboe and piano and singing). It was nearing the end of the first half of the school year, so musical concerts were approaching, and mid-term tests were, too. With the body cast and the reclining wheelchair, I made modifications to attend class, but it was still difficult to do everything, and it took an exaggerated amount of time to get everything accomplished.

Since I was reclining in the wheelchair, I could not push myself around from class to class, so I needed a classmate or friend to push me to where I needed to go. This went well, except when I was pushed to band and choir. The band and choir rooms were located off our only stage at the time, so to get to these classes, we had to walk across the stage. Some of my classmates and "friends," however, thought that it was hilarious to threaten to push me off the stage. They would push me as close to the edge of the stage as possible, let me stare down into the darkness below, and then pretend like they were going to let me go into the fairly deep drop-off. It was terrifying, and I did not want another body cast, but this time it would contain broken bones! In addition, there was a ramp that my classmates had to use to get me up onto the stage. It was a fairly steep ramp, and there was a series of lockers at the end of it. My classmates would also pretend to let me go to the top of the ramp and make me believe that I would fly down the ramp and smash into the lockers.

Ultimately, we discovered that the body cast helped with my pain, and my first back surgery, which consisted of fusing the lumbar spine, was scheduled for St. Patrick's Day 1997, during my senior year of high school. This surgery also involved going in through both the spine and the stomach to fuse the lumbar vertebrae. It was absolutely brutal, and the recovery period was quite long. Part of the reason why the surgery was so brutal is that to fuse my spine, they needed additional bone to do so. Back then, they shaved off a piece of my hip to use, and I have a separate scar just from this part of the surgery. Today, they no longer use this method, but rather, they use cadaver bone to fuse the spine. The reason why they no longer use bone shaved from the hip is that it is so painful to do this both at the time and far into the future, and it can cause a lifetime of pain for the patient. Guess who also has chronic pain where bone was shaved from her hip? If you guessed me, you are correct.

Shortly after the fusion surgery, the surgeon needed to operate again because there was a set of screws that were too close to a nerve. That resulted in numbness and partial paralysis of my right leg, which was a bit terrifying because we did not know if it would be permanent. Once the set of screws was removed, the majority of the numbness, weakness, and partial paralysis was fixed, and I could return to healing from both surgeries. However, I still retained some numbness, tingling, and weakness in the right leg that has only become more pronounced with the additional back surgeries and with time.

Since it was the second half of my senior year of high school, and since I had been announced as the valedictorian of my high school class, my teachers were very kind about giving me homework and tests while I was recovering, which took the remainder of the semester. I still had work to do, but I was also excused from doing a few projects, homework assignments, and tests. I was heartbroken, however, that I was going to miss the band and choir trip to Disney World in Orlando, Florida. I raised money throughout my four years in high school to go on this trip, and both the band and choir would be attending, so a huge part of my class and a great deal of the entire high school were gone during this time. I was at the height of my recovery, and it was a bit depressing because my friends were gone.

I was so excited when everyone returned, and I was honored that some of my friends returned with a gift for me – my name embroidered on Mickey Mouse ears. I was excited to hear all about the trip until I heard some devastating news. My boyfriend during my senior year of high school was my first REAL boyfriend, and we experienced a lot of firsts together. I was madly in love with him, and he even said, "I love you" first. He was a bit younger than I, but he was a tremendous athlete, student, and musician. He was one of the most popular boys from our school, and he was incredibly attractive. During the trip to Florida, however, he started dating another girl, and I had to hear the news from each of my friends who visited or called me to catch up about the Florida trip.

I was devastated by this news. My parents were high school sweethearts, and I had envisioned this path for us, too. Yet, it was not meant to be, and I was very upset and quite depressed with this news. To help cheer me up, my parents, who are always willing to do anything for their children, dressed up in country western gear, and they found some toys and sang me a Faith Hill and Tim McGraw duet. It was hilarious because my dad put a tiny country western Barbie hat on his head, and they both did some hilarious antics during the song.

Eventually, though, I got the last word. I was driving a few years later, and I saw my ex-boyfriend driving around in his Jeep. He told me that he pulled over to a phone booth and found my phone number in a phone book because I had a landline. Everyone had a landline at that time, AND phone booths and phone books really existed! I was at my apartment when he called, and I happened to answer the phone, but I was moving back home for the summer the following day. We talked a little, and he promised to call me just to talk and catch up when I moved back home. He did call, but after we got caught up with each other's lives, he actually asked me out. I had just started dating my husband, however, and we were about two months into the best relationship that I had ever experienced. So, I gently got to let him down this time. It is funny how life works. I was recovering from a major back surgery when I got dumped by this man and found out he had started dating someone else. Yet, I met the love of my life, my husband, while I was recovering from a different back surgery, when he made Valentine's Day dinner for my friend and me. A full circle moment came around when my ex-boyfriend asked me out again, but I could not do that to Troy and our beautiful relationship, so I gently got to let him down.

My recovery from the lumbar fusion back surgery continued through the last day of school for the seniors. Before our final day, I was able to attend a few classes a day, which included both band and choir, because I was the featured Senior Soloist for both. I was also playing and singing in just about every ensemble that was available, and I always felt more comfortable practicing everything. Plus, I was playing a pretty intricate oboe solo with the band, and we needed to coordinate everything with each other. On the final day of my senior year of high school, I forced myself to attend the entire day at school so that I could be with my classmates and experience the same things as they did throughout the day. I also met with a large group of friends at a local restaurant after school was over, and we got to reminisce and just be together without being in school.

The day before graduating from high school, I got laryngitis and could barely talk. We had a dress rehearsal where we rehearsed entering and exiting the gymnasium, and then the valedictorian and salutatorian could practice their speeches. I could not even practice my speech a little bit, which made me nervous; however, I knew that I needed to not talk that day to possibly get my voice back. The next day was both my graduation from high school as well as my 18th birthday, and miraculously, I had my full voice back and was able to give my speech. Due to recovery from my surgery, I required just a little help getting up and down from the stage. I also had to use a pillow on my chair so that I could make it a bit more comfortable through the ceremony. Other than that, my back was completely healed by the time I went to college.

I started college with a major in chemistry and a minor in music, intending to go to pharmacy school after the first two years of college.

Yet, after 1 ½ years of school, I encountered organic chemistry and decided to completely change my major. So, I ended up graduating from college in 3 ½ years with a Bachelor of Science (BS) degree in political science and a minor in sociology. I also graduated with a perfect 4.0 in my major, which helped clarify that I was on the right path. During that final semester, I also studied for the LSATs, which are the entrance exams for law school, and eventually took them. I did okay on the test and ended up getting accepted to Ohio State University, as well as St. Louis University. I ended up choosing St. Louis University because they had the number one healthcare law program in the country, which was the specialty that I thought I wanted to go into.

In between the semester when I graduated from college and the first semester of law school at the beginning of the new academic year, I had back surgery to fuse a portion of my thoracic spine. This allowed me the opportunity to recover during that second half of the academic school year, and I ended up with a paid internship in the legal department at one of our local medical facilities. The project that I did for the medical facility was self-started and self-motivated, and they allowed me to work from home so that I had ample time to recover.

Despite the lumbar fusion and the thoracic fusion, I continued to grow crooked, and I had tremendous bone, muscle, and nerve pain, which you will read about soon. I also determined that both law school and St. Louis were just not for me. St. Louis was a large city, and I was from a town with a population of 1,300. For fun, we went to the "big" city of La Crosse, consisting of around 100,000 people throughout La Crosse and the surrounding area. Furthermore, in law school, they want you to divorce your feelings from everything, and I had a lot of trouble doing that. My heart just was not in it, so I returned home to my family and Troy, and I went back to the school that gave me my undergraduate degree to get my master's in business administration (MBA), which I hoped would be versatile when I graduated and searched for a job. When I did look for a job, I ended up being told that I had too much education and not enough experience, despite my paid internship and the breadth and depth of the work that I did at the Chancellor's Office at the University of Wisconsin-La Crosse during my undergraduate and graduate degrees.

Nevertheless, I accepted a full-time job at an employer that conducted drug testing for large companies. Yet, I was coming home incredibly sore every day, and I also would work throughout the week, but then needed to crash and rest during the weekends. I was not much fun to be around, and it was a terrible way to live, nor could I do much outside of working because I needed the downtime. Eventually, however, I ended up having a terrible accident that forced me to stop working altogether. As I wrote about previously, I fell out of bed and fractured my sacrum. It was extremely painful, and I ended up needing to recover for an entire year on the couch. Thus, I had to take a leave from my job, and my sacrum and lower back have never felt the same way again. Even though the fracture had healed after one year of resting on the couch, the combination of the sacral fracture and the bone that was shaved from my right hip caused me pain every time my right foot took a step down onto whatever surface I was walking on. Each. Step. Was. Excruciating! To take some of the pressure off the right side and to deal with some of the paralysis and weakness, I started walking with a cane in my early to mid-20s, which helped a little because every step I took with my right foot was buffered at least a little bit by the cane.

From the time that I had my first back surgery in 1997 through my final fusion surgery in 2014, I had continuing issues with the pedicle screws in my back. The result was the removal of several sets of pedicle screws once the fusion was stable. The problem was that I had very little tissue through parts of my spine, and this was because when the tumor was removed, a lot of tissue in the surrounding areas was also removed. Furthermore, I had radiation to the spine, and that can leave you with friable scar tissue that is paper-thin. Thus, the instrumentation in my spine would protrude out, and when it was bumped, I had horrific pain and a bone-chilling reaction going up and down my spine. As a result, and several years before my last back surgery, I had all of the instrumentation removed from my spine, as I was told that the fusion was holding incredibly well and this would not affect that.

Throughout my ongoing struggle with chronic back pain, I frequently visited my local medical facility's pain management department. While I sought consultations at a few other pain clinics during my journey from age 14 until now, I consistently returned to my local facility for continuity of care, as I felt I was receiving the best overall treatment there. As you've read, my pain progressively worsened with age, and in 2014, a young neurosurgeon named Dr. Douglas Hughes joined the medical center where I received care. Fortunately, I secured an appointment with him, and he discovered that my spine had become even more crooked. We were astonished, as we believed the fusion surgeries would prevent this. However, Dr. Hughes explained that since the thoracic and lumbar fusions were never joined and fused together, there was enough unfused spine to cause further curvature. I had often wondered about this but hesitated to raise the issue, thinking the surgeons must know best. Additionally, Dr. Hughes suspected that some vertebrae in my back might need to be re-fused due to the increased curvature evident in the scans.

In the summer of 2014, at the age of 35, I had the largest, most difficult fusion surgery of my life. I would be getting my back fused and re-fused from the top of my thoracic spine down to my sacrum. Instrumentation would be put in at every level of the fusion to hold it in place, so my back would once again look like a hardware store. Given all of the levels of fusion and the complexity of the surgery, as well as the physical capacity that it took to contort my back and get it as close to straight as possible, the surgery took 10 hours to complete. Yet, after a grueling surgery, everything went well, and he was happy with the outcome.

I, on the other hand, had a really difficult time waking up from the surgery, and once I did wake up in the Intensive Care Unit (ICU), I was wailing and crying because the pain was so horrific. Given that I regularly take opioids for my chronic back pain, finding pain medicines to treat my pain is always a difficult task, especially after surgery. This is the reason why we have cut back to a small amount of daily opioids for my chronic pain, and we save the stronger opioids for things like surgeries. However, it still can be difficult to stay on top of the pain, and after this intense back surgery, we just could not get ahead of the pain. I remember that my husband, parents, and best friend were really upset seeing me in so much pain, and I felt terrible when I saw the glistening of tears in their eyes. Yet, I also had no control over my reaction as I was waking up from 10+ hours of anesthesia.

I also ended up needing a blood transfusion in the ICU after the surgery. I understand that after operating for so long, I lost a lot of blood and, therefore, became anemic and needed additional blood to catch up and get my body back to its "normal" baseline blood count. This was also not my first blood transfusion, nor would it be my last.

I was initially expected to stay in the hospital for about 4 to 5 days, followed by 1½ weeks of inpatient rehab, also within the hospital. However, physical therapy (PT) and occupational therapy (OT) had me engaging in numerous exercises and modifications early in my recovery. This led to the decision that I was making such significant progress that I no longer needed to enter the inpatient rehab department. I wasn't fully aware that I had the option to decline the PT and OT exercises, and had my family and I understood that participating in them would keep me from inpatient rehab, I might not have been so eager to comply with everything they suggested. Instead of the minimum two weeks, they projected for my hospital stay, I was discharged just 9 days after surgery. While it was fantastic to be home, where I heal best, I felt guilty because my family had to provide more care for me than we had anticipated. If I had gone to inpatient rehab, I would have likely been more independent by the time I returned home, but I never received that chance.

While I was in the hospital, the time came for the medical staff to remove the staples that went from the bottom of my neck down to my butt. We measured the incision, and it was 20 inches long and looked like a long zipper. I knew that it would take quite a bit of time to remove every staple, and we had a bet going as to how many staples would be removed from my back. I do not think that anyone came close to guessing the actual number, except for the intern and me, after things had gotten started. It turned out that I had 100 staples in my back, and it did take quite a while to remove each one. There were times when it was quite easy and not very painful. Then, there were times when there was more sensitivity because of the location of the staple, but it was still not even comparable to the pain I experienced when I woke up after this surgery. After that level of pain, things are really put into perspective!

I had also noticed that after my back surgeries, especially the one in 2014, the area where my neuroblastoma tumor was removed became incredibly painful, even more than the usual severe pain. I always wondered if it was the scarred, radiated tissue adjusting to the new position that my back had been pulled into. Whatever the reason, it was incredibly painful, and I had to be very careful and deliberate with my movements, especially in the hospital when I had just finished the surgery. No one could or would ever give me a reason for this pain, so essentially, I developed my own plausible explanation.

At least one year after the fusion surgery, we started to remove a few levels of instrumentation. In total, we needed to remove two levels on the right side and one level of instrumentation on the left side. The reason for this was that the instrumentation was directly over places where there was little tissue to create a cushion between the skin and the instrumentation. The instrumentation would protrude and become intensely painful, especially if those parts were bumped or hit. And, since those portions stuck out significantly every time I sat on something with a back, those spots would be bumped, and the severe pain would send shivers up and down my spine.

Yet, after those levels were removed, a couple more places with instrumentation started to protrude. It was explained to me by Dr. Hughes, however, that no matter how many levels of instrumentation we removed, the instrumentation below that level would start to stick out and cause pain. I had asked if there was a way to add some fat to that part of my back so that the instrumentation could be somewhat cushioned. Yet, I was informed that there was not enough space within the tissue to even inject some fat cells to help cushion things. So, this was one more pain issue that I needed to just learn to deal with. Although that was incredibly disappointing to hear, I appreciated the honesty rather than trying for something that just was not possible.

The fusion surgery in 2014 was a success because my spine was straightened as much as it could be, and since the fusions had been joined together, the curvature would no longer increase. I also had a few other perks, but the back pain in my bones, muscles, and nerves remained just as bad as it had previously been. Originally, I had hopes that the surgery would help with that, but the medical staff was very careful not to raise my hopes that the pain would decrease or disappear, and I was very thankful for that because the pain levels did not change at all.

Chronic Pain:

Due to my scoliosis and back pain, I have severe limitations in lifting, flexibility, bending, stretching, sitting, standing, and moving, as well as muscle weakness and nerve problems. The most severe condition, however, is my chronic, meaning every minute of every hour, during every day, and severe back pain. I have tried various prescription medications, physical and occupational therapies, cortisone shots, and a menagerie of other methods of possible pain relief, but nothing has eliminated or reduced my symptoms long-term. To help lessen some of the pain and to help with the weakness and numbness on my right side, I walk with a cane for short distances. For longer distances, or when I am expected to be on my feet for extended periods, I use a wheelchair to get around. I have accepted the fact that I will have some level of back pain for the rest of my life, as well as arthritis in my spine. However, I refuse to accept the fact that things will never get better and that, ultimately, things will just continue to worsen as I age. Thus, I am continuously hoping and praying for some sort of improvement, and I continue to try various treatments whenever one is presented.

Unless a person experiences significant chronic pain and its effects, it can be difficult to completely understand it. Even the medical community does not understand how pain, and especially chronic pain, works. Pain is defined as a "localized or generalized unpleasant bodily sensation or complex of sensations that...is characterized by physical discomfort (such as pricking, throbbing, or aching), and...mental and or emotional distress or suffering."

My chronic, bone, muscle, and nerve pain in my back is the late effect that affects me the most. The pain occurs in my neck, upper back, lumbar spine, and sacrum. I also often have constant, severe nerve and muscle pain in the cardiothoracic scar that is a result of the removal of my tumor, due to the scarred, radiated tissue. At times, it feels like my cancer scar is slowly, painfully ripping open. Furthermore, I have neuropathy and weakness in my right leg, so, along with the pain, these medical conditions require me to walk with a cane and use a wheelchair for long distances. I also work with a pain clinic and take regular opioids, as well as prescription medications for muscle and nerve pain. Due to this, I have a high tolerance for opioids, and it is very difficult to find medications that work effectively to dull the pain. Thus, I need a "cocktail" of medications to address the different types of pain.

Although it is extremely difficult, if not virtually impossible, to describe chronic pain, I am going to attempt to detail a cursory explanation. In my case, I experience bone, muscle, and nerve pain, so I have a host of "sensations" that are characterized not only by pricking, throbbing, and aching but also by stabbing, "pins and needles," and burning. My pain begins with a general ache, and my bones and joints are also very stiff and arthritic. Yet, due to activity, fatigue, and stress, the pain progresses throughout the day to intense sharpness and extreme pain. The pain sears throughout my tissues, and it feels like my old cancer and back fusion scars are painfully ripping open and tearing apart. The muscles surrounding my bones start to spasm, and that, in turn, causes me to writhe in agony, misery, and distress. It also pierces and penetrates throughout my skin, muscles, tissues, and bones. My pain is constant and unwavering, and it increases throughout the day because I am doing more and more, no matter how much I try to limit myself. Yet, there is always a baseline, nagging pain that is always present. Furthermore, without any reprieve from the pain, I can get frustrated, exhausted, and, at times, angry from the persistent torture.

It may seem that the physical sensations and characteristics at work are the sole components of chronic pain; however, the worst part may be the emotional turmoil. Since the symptoms of chronic pain have the potential to overtake my life, I try to mask my emotions from others.

This is exhausting, and it has forced me to withhold sharing a small portion of myself with others at times. I desperately try to avoid seeking sympathy and "complaining" about my situation to others. I have seen firsthand that people do not want to be around those who constantly discuss or complain about their medical issues. A high school friend used to tell anyone who would listen about her medical situation with her knee, and I eventually saw my classmates go out of their way to avoid her at all possible costs so that they would not have to listen to her. Upon observing this, I vowed never to sound like my classmate and would try to avoid becoming like her. Yet, there are times when I need to talk to someone about my medical issues, and I do have some wonderful people in my life whom I can go to for this. Yet, there is a fine line between asking for advice and sounding like you are complaining, and this can take an emotional toll on all of those involved.

My high school friend often exaggerated minor issues, much like the boy who repeatedly cried, "Wolf." When he truly needed help, no one believed him, and his concerns were overlooked. His constant embellishments caused him to lose the trust and support of the townspeople, a trust that is nearly impossible to regain. Similarly, my friend faced several knee surgeries, but she made such a fuss each time that after the initial surgeries, my classmates grew disinterested in offering her the extra attention she sought. They felt she had cried "surgery" too often. Given the number of surgeries I've had in the past and continue to have, I am very mindful of how I present these experiences and seek attention for them. I usually try to incorporate humor when discussing my medical challenges, as I believe it makes the topic more relatable and engaging.

Experiencing pain evokes a whirlwind of emotions, predominantly feelings of pessimism, depression, anger, and unhappiness. As someone living with chronic pain, I find this journey to be mentally and emotionally draining, as it is a constant presence in my life. I wake up with pain and go to bed with it, and throughout the day, it intensifies, leaving me feeling utterly exhausted, both mentally and physically. Getting through the day is a challenge, and I must take time to rest and rely on medication to manage the bone, muscle, and nerve pain. To be a person others enjoy being around, I often force a smile and pretend that everything is fine. However, maintaining this façade is incredibly tiring, and by the end of the school or workday, I have little energy left for social activities. Furthermore, a definitive "cure" for chronic pain remains elusive for scientists, medical professionals, and those of us affected by it. While various treatments may provide temporary relief, I often find that their effects last only a few hours. Consequently, I sometimes feel completely hopeless and depressed. The thought of enduring this pain for the rest of my life is frightening, and I often question my ability to cope, especially if it continues to escalate. Thus, during the most intense moments of pain, holding onto hope for the future can be a struggle; however, it is indeed achievable, and this will be explored in more detail in the third section of this book.

I feel like I have tried almost everything under the sun to help with pain. I have been on trials of medication both before my kidney disease diagnosis, when I could try practically anything, and now, after the diagnosis, when it is a bit more difficult to try certain medications. I have tried pain patches, exercises, yoga, pilates, a TENS unit, nerve stimulation, ice and heat, and natural oils. I have had various injections, years of physical therapy, and pool therapy. I have slept and walked on magnets, worn copper bracelets, and tried biofeedback, meditation, and acupuncture. I have also met with several pain clinics at various prestigious medical institutions, yet I always returned to my local medical facility for pain medicine care.

We also approached the topic of pain control holistically, so I had appointments with a psychologist in behavioral therapy, we addressed my insomnia and tried to ensure that I was getting a good night's sleep, and that I ate a healthy diet. Yet, nothing seemed to help my pain, and it continued to be a huge issue. In my late 20s, a pain pump was proposed to me as a possible solution. The theory is that you no longer need to take any oral pain medications because there is a pump delivering medications right to the fluid surrounding the spinal cord. This was supposed to cut out the need for oral pain medications and all of the potential side effects that come with them. However, I found out that often, patients still had to take oral pain medications even if they had a pain pump. In addition, the dosage of the pump will vary because the body will get used to a particular dose. When that is the case, it is necessary to raise the dosage of the medication coming out of the pain pump. This is all done on a very slow basis, but there is a limit as to how much medication you can get through the pain pump. The pain pump is put into people in their 50s or 60s, or even older. Given that I was only in my late 20s, we would have to keep raising the levels of medication in my drug pump, as well as any oral medications, because I was too young to keep taking a small dosage through the pain pump. In addition, given that I had bone, muscle, and nerve pain, I would likely need to continue taking a muscle relaxer, as well as a prescription for nerve pain.

Yet, the main reason why I did not want to have an intrathecal pain pump implanted in me was that the surgery was incredibly risky. To get the pain pump, a surgeon would need to feed the tube portion of the drug pump down my spine, while carefully avoiding the spinal cord. I guess this was a bit more straightforward for a person who had a straight spine that was not fused. However, we were told by others with "horror stories" that this could be quite difficult for someone with scoliosis that was completely fused, or even partially fused.

I was trying in vain to get this information from my pain doctor and have him see my side of the situation, but he just seemed to want to push ahead with getting the pain pump rather than listening to my concerns. He was pushing so hard, and I felt so pressured that I just had to stop the entire process. At first, my doctor asked if I had stopped the process because I wanted to keep taking oral pain medications! I calmly tried to explain that this was definitely not the reason, but I felt like he was not listening to me, and he was judging me for the decision that I felt like I had to make. Luckily, that doctor was not around for very long, and he ended up leaving that medical facility. Talk about the intrathecal drug pump stopped completely once he left.

My chronic pain began when I was around 14 years old, and each year, it continues to worsen. Unfortunately, as I have mentioned previously, it is expected that the severity and strength of my pain will likely continue to worsen throughout my life, and that is hard to comprehend because the pain feels so strong and insurmountable already. My family and I will continue to pray for new ways to treat chronic pain because it is difficult to imagine worse pain than what I currently have.

My chronic pain has consistently been intense, and from the onset, I have been prescribed various forms of opioid medication to manage it. Having experienced chronic back pain since I was 14, I have been relying on some type of opioids for many years. Before the opioid epidemic, there was a different school of thought among pain doctors regarding opioids. If a certain strength of opioids was not helping with pain control, doctors would just prescribe more opioids. I especially learned that this was true right after I broke my sacrum, and even after my sacrum was healed. I was newly married and in my mid-20s, yet I was a shell of myself and essentially just a bump on the couch. The higher level of opioids also meant that I slept a great deal of the time, and I honestly do not remember much during this time of my life. I was a terrible wife to my husband for some of the early years of our marriage because all I could do was lie on the couch. This was a terrible way to live, and I did not even have great pain management either. A change needed to be made, but it was scary to think about making any changes because, although I did not have much of a life, I did not want to be in increased levels of agony.

A little less than a year after my significant back surgery in 2014, Linda, the nurse practitioner I primarily collaborate with at my local pain clinic, informed me that I needed to embark on a "narcotics holiday." (Just a heads up, when they suggest something, you really don't have a choice and must follow their recommendations!) This particular holiday felt incredibly daunting to me, as it required gradually tapering off the opioids until I was no longer taking any. Following that, I would spend a few months opioid-free to assess whether my pain levels remained the same, improved, or worsened. The main goal of this process was to determine if the opioids were genuinely alleviating some of my pain because, over time, the body can become accustomed to the medication, reducing its overall effectiveness.

The opioid holiday was both the worst and the best time in my life for completely different reasons. It was the worst time because tapering down the opioids was accidentally done too fast, and I experienced severe withdrawal symptoms. I was balled up on the floor in blankets because I was cold, yet my body was also hot and sweating at the same time. I was extremely nauseous and dizzy, and I had a "puke pail" next to me to use when my head was not hanging over the toilet. Every minute of the clock ticking by felt like agony, and time seemed to almost stand still and take forever. Honestly, all that I wanted was just to fall asleep so that I could avoid hours of being awake and experiencing the withdrawal symptoms, but I could only lie there with my eyes wide open, struggling through each minute on the clock that was slowly ticking by directly in front of me. I could not concentrate on anything but that clock, and trying not to jump out of my skin because I was so miserable and uncomfortable. I also could not do anything else to help pass the time because I felt that horrific. I was also in extreme pain throughout my back, sacrum, and cancer scar. The couch felt too confining, so I would lie writhing on the floor in agony, pain, and discomfort.

The experience was incredibly challenging, yet it seems it shouldn't have been that difficult. Initially, the process of tapering off the opioid was meant to be gradual and careful, but I was tapered down far too quickly, resulting in withdrawal symptoms. During my next appointment with the pain management team, they informed me that I should have expressed how much I was struggling, as there was a medication available to ease the transition. After adjusting the tapering schedule of the opioids and beginning the new medication to help with the withdrawal symptoms, things improved somewhat. While it wasn't enjoyable or entirely comfortable, I was at least able to get through the day and accomplish a few tasks.

You may be asking yourself how this could have possibly been one of the best times of my life, considering how horrible the opioid holiday had started. Once I was off the opioids completely and there were no more symptoms of withdrawal, it was almost as if I awoke from a LONG slumber, similar to Sleeping Beauty or Snow White after she ate the poisonous apple. I was no longer that bump on the couch, and I started becoming more active in life. This is also the time when I started becoming involved in childhood cancer nonprofits, and that work truly fulfills me and gives me purpose, joy, and drive. It is my life's work, and you will read more about that in the next section of this book. Overall, I am so thankful that I was able to become clear-headed and start working with the Neuroblastoma Children's Cancer Society (NCCS), which gave me a home and a place to start all of my nonprofit work.

Although I thoroughly enjoyed and took advantage of finally being awake and able to participate in life as a fully functioning human being, I was in a severe amount of chronic back pain throughout the three months that I was completely off opioids. This likely told us that the opioids had been working for me, and they would continue to work for me. Once three months without any opioids had passed, the holiday that no one ever wants to take was over, and I was put on a small dose of extended-release opioids that we could tailor a bit to help take the edge off my pain. However, we discussed the fact that I would never again want to live as I had been living, which was on the couch in a complete fog. I wanted to remain awake and engaged in the world, working with childhood cancer nonprofits. I also wanted my family to continue "having Mariah back" because they deserved more than what I had been able to give while I was on high levels of opioids. I am thankful, however, that I can still take a small dose of this medication to help take the edge off the pain while still being alert, bright-eyed, and engaged with the world.

My pain and medical issues continue to affect my everyday life, and the most frustrating aspect is how they interfere with my activities and aspirations, particularly regarding my nonprofit work. I have a deep passion for what I do and am receiving incredible opportunities in the childhood cancer community, where I can assist patients, families, and survivors. However, I find myself physically and medically unable to take full advantage of all these wonderful chances. Accepting this reality is incredibly challenging for me, yet it doesn't always stop me from making an effort. Consequently, I often overwork myself, neglecting self-care and failing to take sufficient time off to rest. This not only exacerbates my pain but also intensifies my other medical conditions. The irony lies in the fact that engaging in this work fills my heart and soul, providing me with a sense of purpose and value, which is crucial. I am uncertain if I will ever master this balance, but I am determined to keep trying.

Additionally, chronic pain often leads to feelings of loneliness, and the weight of that can be both frightening and depressing. When I find myself feeling isolated, I typically seek a way to connect with someone. However, there are times when it feels nearly impossible to find comfort and solace. Just when I think I can't endure it any longer, a stranger unexpectedly enters my life, offering support that helps lift my spirits and, more importantly, helps me gain perspective at precisely the right moment. For instance, I once had a doctor's appointment where I received the devastating news that I would be living with severe, chronic back pain for the rest of my life. To make matters worse, the doctor informed me that there were no treatments available to alleviate the pain. Hearing such news is incredibly difficult, and emotions like sadness, anger, and frustration rise to the surface, prompting me to fight back tears. In addition, I often find myself grappling with a "feeling sorry for myself" mindset, accompanied by emotions of loss, abandonment, and loneliness. I truly despise it when I start to wallow in self-pity, and I strive to resist these feelings for as long as possible. It feels like I'm at my lowest point when suddenly, God provides me with a miraculous sign to uplift my spirits. This sign often takes the form of someone visibly struggling with a medical condition even more severe than my own. I am certain these individuals also experience feelings of isolation, loss, and abandonment, yet they persevere. Witnessing them live their lives inspires me to keep moving forward and to express gratitude for the blessings I have received.

Although acute pain may be treated and alleviated with analgesics, such as ibuprofen or acetaminophen, or prescriptions for a short length of time, chronic pain involves a combination of physical rehabilitation, psychological support, and medication over long periods. However, it is also entirely possible for chronic pain to be untreatable. Therefore, many sufferers of chronic pain, including myself, are left with the devastating symptoms of pain for which there are little to no treatments to alleviate it.

You may remember that my chronic back pain started when I was around 14 after we removed my back brace, and I ripped and sprained my back muscles because I was trying to be a golfer. After that, and after several back surgeries, my pain continued to worsen. Each year, I would notice that I would hurt a bit more. We searched for answers to this pain, but my back was fairly messed up from the radiation, the curvature of my spine continued to become more severe, and multiple spinal issues were going on with my bones, muscles, and nerves. We did not want someone to just do surgery on my back, but we wanted a holistic approach that treated everything.

One day, when I was about 19 years old, I saw my back doctors, otherwise known as my orthopedic surgeons, at the Mayo Clinic. I was going to take myself to this appointment because it was just a check-up, but for some reason, possibly divine intervention, my parents insisted that my brother go with me, too. This doctor and his staff had always been so confident and positive about things in the past, but that day during my appointment, he came into the office and told me that I would continue to have back pain throughout the rest of my life. I said that I knew that was a possibility, but he continued by saying that I would always have back pain, and there was nothing that really could be done about it, and it would just continue to worsen as I grew older.

Those statements hit me like a ton of bricks and took the air out of both me and the room. I am not sure how I got from that room to my car without losing it, but my brother, even though he was only about 14 years old at the time, got the gravity of the situation and was quite worried about me. Getting to the car without a reaction, however, almost gave him false hope that I was okay after the appointment. Yet, when we finally got to the car, I lost it and started crying because each of those statements was utterly devastating to me. I did not always want back pain, and I could not even fathom this because I was so young and had felt like I had so much life to live. Also, to know that there was likely nothing that could be done about my pain and that it would continue to worsen as I got older seemed extra cruel and unusual. I could not stop crying, but my little brother just sat there, patted my hand, and listened to me. Listening, sitting still, and not talking were usually not his strongest characteristics, but he was incredibly mature as I reacted to this news. He then leaned over and hugged me, and it truly did help. I was so glad to have him there with me at this appointment. Sitting in my car in the Mayo Clinic parking garage with my brother comforting me is a memory that I will never forget, and it was an important bonding moment between us.

When I married my husband, Troy, I had chronic pain, but I was still able to work outside of the home, and I had not yet broken my sacrum. I had just finished school and was searching for my "grown-up" full-time job. Yet, as our marriage progressed, my medical conditions and chronic pain worsened to the point where I have not been able to do much outside of the home. I feel so bad that I have not been able to attend different events with Troy, and it saddens me that I cannot go and that he is there alone without me. I know that it is probably difficult to explain to people why I am not there, but it is important to me that Troy knows that I wish I could be there with him. I have fears that I will be like this forever or that things will continue to decline and the pain will continue to increase, resulting in my being on the couch more and more. I hope that this is not the case because I want to be a better, more present wife. Furthermore, I feel terrible that I cannot financially contribute to our family anymore with a full-time professional salary, using the education that I was so blessed to receive and the degrees that I so carefully studied for and obtained. Eventually, I did qualify for Social Security Disability

Income (SSDI), so I felt a bit better that I could contribute something to our finances.

My medical conditions also make many regular household chores difficult, but Troy cooks, cleans, and does the laundry happily and without complaint. I am quite OCD about a clean house, so I do everything that I absolutely can to keep the house clean. I rest so much better in a clean house, and I want to do as much as I can to contribute to the household chores. There are some chores that I just cannot do, however, so that is when Troy comes in. In addition to working full-time, he also does most of the grocery and household shopping, and he patiently and kindly fetches things for me when I am lying on the couch with a cat on top of me. I always try to let him know how grateful and appreciative I am for all that he does.

Unfortunately, most people do not know that childhood cancer survivors deal with the ramifications of their cancer and its treatments every day, even after treatment has ended. Just because treatment ended does not mean that childhood cancer has ended. Childhood cancer does not simply occur during childhood; survivors also deal with it during adulthood, as well. Most people do not know this, and if they do, they may not understand the severity of the late effects and other medical issues that plague childhood cancer survivors. Part of the reason is that most people have never experienced a serious medical issue in their lives, so it is impossible for them to even know about or understand the situation. Also, I once heard that those living with chronic pain or another chronic condition feel like they are misunderstood, and they may not have anyone that they can talk to who will truly listen, understand, and accept them. This is incredibly sad, and since that time, I have really made an extra effort to appreciate and value the people in my life whom I can talk to for advice.

I also recognize that most of the population does not understand what it is like to be a childhood cancer survivor living with the effects of an illness that some of us barely even remember. Yet, childhood cancer and its treatments are so brutal and toxic that they can affect us for the rest of our lives. It can also affect some of us more than others, and we live every day for the rest of our lives with the effects of childhood cancer and the many chronic medical conditions that accompany survivorship. Believe it or not, this misunderstanding does not simply apply to strangers; rather, I have family and loved ones who essentially refuse to acknowledge that I have medical conditions. They do not check in with me by phone or in person, and they really have no interest in wanting to know how I am doing or what is currently happening with my various medical conditions. I fully understand that sometimes people are not comfortable discussing medical issues, especially if they are not close to you. Although the work that I do is related to my medical background, I do have many other areas of interest that I can discuss with them. I am not sure if people are just afraid to talk to me because they might have to confront negative feelings and/or think about personal medical issues, but I do not talk about them unless I am specifically asked. There are so many medical issues that I have never discussed, and I was raised not to talk about them.

Secondary Cancers and Cancer Scares

You may remember that Dr. Mutter was the radiation oncologist that Troy and I saw in December 2017, in part to see if I needed to have a prophylactic mastectomy on the right side of my chest. Up until that point, I was only aware of a few secondary cancers that I was at a higher risk of contracting. Because I had radiation to the chest and I had an anthracycline chemotherapy medication, we had already discussed the fact that breast cancer was a high risk for me. I was advised, for example, to have a bilateral mastectomy because before this surgery, Dr. Mutter estimated that I had a 50-85% chance of developing breast cancer.

Additionally, Dr. Mutter estimated that given the age at which I was diagnosed with neuroblastoma, as well as the treatments that I received, my estimated annual risk was similar to a patient with the BRCA 1 or BRCA 2 gene mutation. Furthermore, I could not have additional radiation to my chest because I already had chest radiation with my neuroblastoma treatments. Thus, if I were ever diagnosed with breast cancer, it would need to be found early for me to survive because I could not have radiation to the chest again. Dr. Mutter let us know that a double-sided mastectomy was reasonable to consider, which meant that I would still need to have a mastectomy on the right side. I followed through with that recommendation, and it turns out that I made the right choice because they removed a benign tumor on the left side that could have become cancerous; however, my mammogram had not picked it up, only two months before.

Throughout my life, including my appointment with Dr. Mutter, I was informed that there were no comparable studies on older neuroblastoma survivors who were usually diagnosed and treated between infancy and five years of age. For instance, to understand the likelihood, comparison, and risk of developing breast cancer due to radiation and chemotherapy, data would be gathered from studies on Hodgkin's lymphoma patients, who are typically diagnosed and treated during their teenage years. This highlights that not only are the cancers distinct, but the timing of treatment for the survivors is also vastly different.

I had heard different versions of this before, and I often wondered why and asked if they could use me to start or contribute to these studies during my childhood and adulthood. My goal was never to benefit myself in any way, but I felt like I had a responsibility to help present and future neuroblastoma survivors who had thoracic tumors and were treated in similar ways. I did not want them to go through the uncertainty of learning about late effects as they experienced them, like I had for the first few decades of my life. Neuroblastoma patients, survivors, and their families deserve to know about potential late effects and how to screen, diagnose, and treat them. Furthermore, they deserve to know any information about the risks of secondary cancers and the best screening methods to discover any malignancies early, or to diagnose other late effects in the early stages. I would have gladly joined, contributed, and participated in any type of medical study or discussions.

Another cancer that I was at a high risk of contracting because of the radiation field was thyroid cancer. I say "was" because my risk of contracting thyroid cancer has been mitigated. You may remember that my thyroid had been covered in nodules, and the entirety of it all was pushing against my trachea, so the collective decision was to remove the thyroid and the attached nodules.

Dr. Mutter also told Troy and me about some additional secondary cancers that we had never been aware of before. Another relatively high-risk secondary cancer I had to monitor, with regular visits to a dermatologist, was non-melanoma skin cancer, particularly in areas exposed to radiation. I have established myself with a dermatologist that I see regularly, and he checks my body over once a year for any signs of skin cancer. Additionally, one of the chemotherapy medications that I had can cause bladder cancer, but screening for this is fairly straightforward and involves submitting a yearly urine sample to the lab for a urine cytology test.

There are also some additional secondary cancers that I have a higher risk of getting, but the risk is smaller than the previously discussed cancers. For example, I am at a slightly higher risk of developing different types of leukemias and sarcomas. Also, my right lung was in the radiation field, so as I age, I need to monitor it because I have a higher risk of developing lung cancer. My esophagus was also within the radiation field, so we needed to watch for esophageal cancer. Finally, you also read about my risk of developing colon cancer. It is difficult to determine whether my higher risk of developing colon cancer is a result of my family history, a result of my neuroblastoma treatments, or a combination of the two. Whatever the case may be, I need to have regular colonoscopies, either yearly or every other year, so that the numerous precancerous polyps can be identified and removed.

The reality is that I have had many cancer scares throughout my life, including the ultimate scare of neuroblastoma recurrences, both in my childhood and adulthood. I undergo screening/testing each year for many possible secondary cancers from my treatments, and these will simply increase as I get older. At times, I feel like this is just my reality and just one more test that I need to do, that is really no big deal, because the result is probably negative. Yet, it can also be extremely scary and frightening to think about the possibility of having cancer again, despite how many cancer scares I have experienced.

Despite being pronounced cancer-free at 8 years old, there are still worries that my old cancer, or a new one, could return. I have developed several lumps throughout my life, and immediately, my family and I fear that I will have cancer again because that is just the reality for a cancer survivor. I remember the first lump that I discovered in my body. I was at an awards program for the final week of my Sunday school church program, and I was in elementary school. Coincidentally, it was also my birthday on the same day, and I was preoccupied and distracted from the awards program. I was anxious to begin my birthday party, but was trying to appear as though I was paying attention to the program. I was next to my dad, and I started feeling around my neck, near where my glands were. I then discovered two lumps that were mobile and located on both sides of my neck. I immediately started tearing up, and I went to my dad and asked him if we could talk privately. He saw the fear in my eyes, and we went to the back of our church, where I showed him my lumps. Luckily, after he inspected my neck, my father informed me that the lumps were only lymph nodes and that I had nothing to worry about. I was so thankful that nothing was wrong and that my cancer had not returned, but the fear of recurring cancer was not new to my parents. They had felt that fear ever since I was first diagnosed.

Unfortunately, finding the swollen lymph nodes in my neck was not my last experience with strange lumps. It seemed that whenever a medical problem arose, such as my paralytic arm, the first suspect was cancer, and although it was a recurring theme, we certainly did not get used to the fear.

Towards the end of college, I discovered a lump at the base of my spine, and immediately, it became worrisome. At the time of discovery, the lump was quite painful, and it became difficult to sit properly without intense pain. A few days after we discovered the lump, we discovered a change in its status. Now, I am sure that you know that any change in size, volume, and/or texture of any lump immediately becomes worrisome. Due to its placement and flexibility limitations, I had to enlist the help of my mom to examine the lump. So, when the lump began oozing, we determined that it was infected. I was supposed to be having minor back surgery within the next few days, but due to the infection near my lower spine, the surgery had to be postponed. We saw a specialist who determined that the lump was a pilonidal cyst, which is simply a non-cancerous collection of cells that develops near the base of the spine. The treatment was to remove the cyst through surgery and then begin a course of antibiotics to keep the surgical area free from infection. After the cyst was removed, I had a hole in my body where it had been. This hole had to heal from the inside to the outside. For that to happen, my mother had to insert sterilized gauze into the surgical "hole" twice daily. Eventually, the skin would grow and "fill in" the hole until there was only a slight scar remaining. Typically, these cysts usually are recurring and will grow back, but so far I have not had any additional problems, and I am hopeful that the surgeon removed all of the cyst, the cyst sac, and the surrounding tissue.

The cyst was removed at the base of my spine in the summer of 2001, and shortly after that problem had been addressed, I discovered another lump on my shoulder, which grew rather quickly. Although we were immediately concerned that the lump could be cancerous, we also thought that perhaps it was just another non-cancerous cyst that needed to be removed. The doctors could not determine what this lump was, however, so they suggested that we have it removed and then test it from there to see if we could determine its origin. The doctors believed it was just another cyst, but after its removal, we discovered that the lump was a misplaced, inflamed lymph node. This node had the possibility of becoming cancerous, or it could already be cancerous, due to its misplacement, growth, and firmness. This was extremely scary to us because cancer of the lymph nodes is difficult to treat, and since I already had cancer treatments as a child, additional steps to treat a tumor may not be as effective or may not even be viable options. Luckily, laboratory tests confirmed that the lymph node was benign, and its removal would ensure that it would not become cancerous.

I think that my most petrifying "cancer scare," however, was one that should have never happened. I cannot quite remember why, but I had to have some X-rays done when I was in college, and since it was no big deal, I went alone to complete the tests, just like I had so many times before. Yet, this time would be quite different and a big deal because after the scans were completed, the X-ray technician told me that my scans showed that my neuroblastoma had returned. I was devastated and shocked, but my biggest fear and concern was calling my mom and telling her about what I had just learned. At the time, I did not even think about why the technician would be telling me this because he was not qualified to do so. I felt so alone, and I was crying, but I got to my car in the parking lot and made that difficult telephone call to my mother to tell her that my neuroblastoma had returned. She screamed, "No," and wailed into the telephone. The sound was deafening and ripped through my heart. I believe that I drove to the school where my mom was employed, and we comforted each other. My dad joined us shortly thereafter, which brought on more tears, hugs, and prayers.

Once we composed ourselves, we called my doctor and got an appointment immediately. Both my parents and I went to that appointment, and we found out that there was nothing to worry about and that whatever "mass" the technician thought he saw was actually what my normal scans always looked like. We talked with someone in hospital administration about my experience to stop the technician from misinforming someone else, and we were assured that he would be talked to and reprimanded in some capacity. I was concerned about "tattling" on the technician, but I was more concerned that he could do this in the future to someone else. What if this person were so upset about this news that they could have a panic attack, exacerbate mental health issues, or even have a heart attack? I never found out what happened to that technician, but he gave us quite a scare, and we never wanted to relive a moment like that again.

Miscellaneous
<u>My Hard Head</u>:

Not all of my secondary medical issues have been from the cancer treatments, and some could even be construed as quite humorous. For example, I seem to have developed an extremely hard head, and my hard head has saved me numerous times. The first time was when I was around eight years old, and I was riding my bike down a gravel path to meet my dad, who was coming home from a long day of work and coaching basketball practice. I got a little overconfident on the gravel, and I turned a corner too hard, wiped out, and gouged open my forehead. I did not cry and was not even really aware that I had injured myself until I saw the blood out of the corner of my eye. When I fell, my dad had just pulled into the driveway and witnessed my spill. He ran out of the car to hug me, and I was upset because I had gotten blood on his shirt. The cut was pretty deep, and we had to go to the ER to get stitches. Luckily, however, I did not have a concussion or anything more sinister than a few stitches to close my forehead, and I still bear the scars from that injury today.

My head also saved me another time...in choir. People find it very humorous and unlikely that I got a concussion in choir, but I managed to do so. In the choir room, the chairs were set up on risers so that we sang on multiple levels and made the best use of the space that we had. One day, without realizing it, I placed my chair so that two legs were hanging off the edge of the riser. The moment I sat down, the chair tipped forward, sending me headfirst into a metal filing cabinet, which I somehow managed to dent with my head. I also got a spectacular bump on the head, as well as angry, large bruises where I fell on my left thigh.

Before my first back fusion surgery, you read that I had to wear a body cast for about ten days, and although many people may halt their lives and stay at home, I continued with school and extracurricular activities. During this time, I had rehearsals for an opera at a local university, and I was hired to play in the pit orchestra with local professional musicians. I could not sit in the body cast, so I had a reclining wheelchair for the classroom. However, the wheelchair could not fit in the orchestra pit, so I had to bring a stool down there to perch on the edge. It was working fairly well until I dropped my pencil. Momentarily, I had forgotten about my cumbersome body cast, and I reached down to pick up my pencil.

When my body could not bend, I fell off balance and started falling headfirst. One of the violin players saw me falling, and he quickly grabbed my oboe before it went down with me. I ended up hitting my head on a music stand, but at least I knew that my oboe was okay! There was another time when my oboe took precedence over my head. I was at a music competition and I almost fainted. I started to slide out of my chair at the end of my performance, and my mom ran forward to grab the expensive oboe, rather than my head. It is a good thing that I have a hard head because my oboe ranks higher than my head. And rightly so!

The most intense head trauma experience I encountered occurred during my first vacation with my husband's family. We attended a Major League Baseball (MLB) game featuring the Milwaukee Brewers and the Minnesota Twins. After enjoying some delicious grilled food while tailgating in the parking lot, we entered Miller Park, as it was known at that time, early enough to catch batting practice. Many fans were eager to snag the baseballs soaring into the outfield, which were coming close to where we were seated. My sister-in-law, Anna, and I decided to move closer to the area where the balls were landing, hoping to catch one (Truthfully, we were also excited to see how cute the players in the outfield were!) However, we were informed that no more balls would be hit, as preparations were underway for the game. Disappointed, we began to walk back up the bleachers to our seats. Just as I turned around for one last look at the field, I was unexpectedly struck on the head and fell onto the ground.

When I was aware again, I realized that Anna was holding me up, and people were swarming around me. A line drive had hit me on the head, directly over the orbital bone of my upper right eye and my forehead, without even bouncing first. I had passed out for a bit, and I was getting a huge bump directly where I had been hit, so a smart, fast-thinking bystander gave me an ice pack from her cooler (this was before 9/11, when coolers were still allowed into the ballpark). The Miller Park ambulance came to get me because I had gotten smacked near an eye orbit, and people were quite concerned that I had fractured something. I appeared to be okay, and the Miller Park doctors told me I should go to the emergency room for X-rays and tests to see if I had suffered a concussion and/or a fracture. I felt horrible, however, that I had already interrupted our vacation and time at the game, so I insisted that we stay for the whole game. I iced throughout the game and felt like passing out, but we stayed until the 8th inning because the Brewers were getting their butts kicked, and Troy's parents wanted me to get checked out.

We visited the emergency room, and thankfully, there were no fractures; however, I did sustain a mild concussion. Thanks to the quick action of a woman with an ice pack, I managed to avoid an impressive black eye. I now have a permanent dent where the ball struck me near my right eyebrow. This serves as a constant reminder, along with the realization that getting hit in a massive stadium feels akin to being struck by lightning or winning the lottery, which I would have much preferred. The most frustrating part was that someone had taken the ball that had hit me, and they refused to return it. The staff at Miller Park kindly compensated me with a World Series ball from the previous year, but alas, that one didn't leave a memorable dent in my head.

Ankle Saga:

Somehow, I managed to fracture the navicular bone of my right ankle sometime between May and August 2023. Apparently, this bone is incredibly strong and difficult to fracture, yet I had managed to fracture it without knowing how I had injured it in the first place. I had taken a picture of my swollen ankle in May, and the broken ankle was diagnosed in August, so I injured it sometime between May and August. My swollen, painful ankle was discovered when I went in for a completely unrelated surgery in early August. The swelling was quite monumental, and to be honest, I had so much swelling that it looked like I had a golf ball-sized protrusion coming out of my ankle. Since I had that scheduled surgery that I had been waiting months for, I decided that I would proceed with the surgery and then take care of the ankle later. Furthermore, my ankle was far enough away from the surgical site, and I did not think that it would impact the surgery.

I checked in for my scheduled surgery, and when the nurse tried to put the compression stockings on my right foot, I tried to explain the situation to her and relay that the swelling was new and I knew that I needed to take care of it, but that I had not been able to at that point. She peeled back the blankets, her eyes widened, and she went to get another nurse to consult and look at it. I was told that my surgery might not happen, but my surgeon had no problem with it because the surgery was located near a region of the body that was unaffected by the fractured, swollen ankle. The nurses did tell me, however, that after I was released from this surgery, I either needed to make an appointment with my general doctor to look at my swollen ankle or go to Urgent Care immediately. My doctor's next open appointment was in three months, so the decision was made for me. I had surgery in the morning, and then I was in Urgent Care in the afternoon.

At Urgent Care, I found out that I fractured the navicular bone in my right ankle, and I was told that I would need to stay in a boot and try to be as non-weight-bearing as possible. This would be difficult for me to do with my existing disabilities and modifications, but I used my walker as much as possible. Yet, little did I know that this ankle fracture would lead to multiple surgeries and many months of issues and recovery. The navicular bone connects the ankle to the bones in our foot, and it also helps form the arch of our foot. The podiatrist I saw told me that it is extremely difficult to fracture this bone because it is quite strong;

however, the navicular bone is prone to stress fractures, specifically from athletes who perform repetitive motions, such as kicking, sprinting, twisting, or falling. Anyone who knows me, however, knows that I am far from being an athlete, so we still cannot identify how and why I fractured my ankle. The only difference that I made the day before was a walk around the block to kick off a new exercise routine. I also did my physical therapy exercises, which I had started several months before the injury. These consisted of exercises meant to strengthen my legs and ankles, and they should not have injured my navicular bone in any way.

Repetitive motions can also cause the bone to break, so perhaps it happened because I ride a recumbent bike for exercise. Or, due to my back issues and the use of a cane, I walk with a significant limp, and I sort of drag my right leg along. Alternatively, there was also talk about my neuroblastoma, the treatments that I had for it, and the possibility that I could have low bone density and maybe progressed from osteopenia to osteoporosis, which could have meant that my bones were weak and could fracture more easily.

I wore a boot faithfully for several months, but I was never able to stay off my foot completely because of my pre-existing back issues. Whether or not this affected me negatively is unknown, but I did my best. Initially, I tried to use crutches to be non-weight bearing, but I almost hurt myself even worse because I was so unsteady and would almost fall. Or, I would start to tip over, and my husband would catch me, but only if he was home. Instead, I tried walking in the modified way that I was taught, on my heels, and I used the walker. This went on for quite a while, and I wore the boot until my doctor told me I could stop, which ended up being in early November. Presumably, I should have been healed by that point, but I was still having lots of pain and swelling.

I was scheduled for a CT Scan in November, directly before Thanksgiving, to see if things were healing. The results were quite shocking and disappointing. The podiatrist informed me that the navicular bone had not healed at all and that I needed to wear the brace again. He also said that I would need surgery to repair the fracture, which involved putting in a staple to close it. I had this surgery on December 8, and it was a successful operation.

Throughout the month of December, I would meet with one of the podiatrists in that department, and they would check everything over to be sure that things were healing properly. My surgeon was out of the office until later in December, so I did not see him during these initial check-ups. Early on, this area was quite swollen, and it became more and more pink as the weeks progressed. It became so bad that I was treated with antibiotics for cellulitis, which is a bacterial skin infection. Things became progressively worse, however, and the antibiotics cleared up nothing. The pink around the incision increased, and there was a slight opening in the incision, which had already been sewn shut and should have been healing.

On January 2, I had an appointment with the podiatrist who performed my surgery, and we shared our concerns with him about a possible infection. As we were talking, they were removing the bandages, and the mood was light and playful. Once the bandages were removed and the surgeon looked at the wound, the light, playful mood disappeared, and you could tell that things became quite serious. The doctor asked for a probe to further investigate that area, and that part of the incision opened up into a large hole. It almost looked like there was black inside there, but that hole just kept on opening. (That evening, we had to change the bandage, and we were SHOCKED at the gaping hole that the wound had opened into. I am typically fine with medical things, but looking at the wound in this state was disgusting.) I was informed that I had developed an infection, and typically, there was only about a 1% chance that an infection would develop after surgery. It was determined that I needed to have surgery as soon as possible to clean out the infection and restart the healing process. I went to the doctor on a Monday, and the surgery was scheduled for that Friday.

In the meantime, we were told how to bandage the wound, and that process became a bit too much for my poor husband to handle. I ended up doing it on my own, and then he would help wrap up my wound after it was covered in various gauze and bandages to protect it. It looked awful and just continued to look worse as the week went on. Luckily, I did not have long to wait because, on Friday, January 5, I had surgery to clean out the massive infection that was in my ankle and foot. The infection was cleaned out as much as possible, and the staple that was used to repair the fracture was removed. In addition, the podiatrist/surgeon used a Wound VAC (Vacuum-Assisted Closure) to help with the healing of the gaping hole in my ankle. The wound vac, as it is also referred to, uses negative wound pressure therapy (NWPT) because when it is turned on, it creates a gentle suction that: removes excess fluid; reduces bacteria; improves blood flow; encourages growth of repair tissue; pulls wound edges together; and stabilizes the wound.

Once I was discharged from the hospital, I had to go to the Wound Clinic for dressing changes three days a week. During the first month of using the Wound VAC and receiving three dressing changes per week at the wound clinic, progress was incredibly slow. First, the wound was large, and it was a bit difficult to think that a wound this size could close on its own. Also, the edges of the wound were macerated and broken down, and there was too much moisture for healing to occur immediately. Furthermore, underneath my skin, I had severe tunneling in a couple of places, which means that the hole in my ankle now extended to form an opening underneath the surface of the skin. This can be very difficult to heal, but even more difficult and quite painful was the fact that I had a huge tendon and nerve running alongside the tunneling. You could see the tendon and the nerve moving when this area was exposed and the hole was open. At times, the nerve felt out of control, and I would get strange and painful sensations. Since this nerve is a large one that feeds areas throughout the foot, it is odd and a bit unnerving to feel sensations from my ankle to my toes. The tendon, however, causes even more pain because that is more exposed. The result is that I have a lot of pain in the front of my ankle, almost like it is severely sprained, but I also feel like I have extreme shin splints.

On Valentine's Day, 2024, my husband and I had a date at 6:15 p.m. with a CT machine. It was around that time that I needed a CT scan to confirm if there was any bone infection, and if there was, I would require immediate treatment. The only available time was either 6:15 a.m. or 6:15 p.m., and my husband and I are not morning people. It was important to get this test done as soon as possible, so that is why we spent our Valentine's evening at our local medical center. And ultimately, we received good news because it was confirmed that there was no bone infection. YAY! Yet, I found out that I somehow broke another bone. I had been in a boot since August when I first learned that I had fractured the navicular bone, but I somehow also fractured one of the three bones that were directly below the navicular bone. The fracture was in the middle of those three bones, called the intermediate cuneiform bone. It is possible that this bone was also fractured when we first discovered that the navicular bone was fractured; however, the fracture of the intermediate cuneiform bone did not show up on the original scans in August, and it was still fractured when the Valentine's Day CT was taken, six months after the original fracture was found.

Very s-l-o-w-l-y, over many months, the hole in my ankle healed. It was so slow that we had scheduled surgery to close the hole because it seemed like things would never fully close on their own. Yet, between the time when we scheduled the surgery and my pre-op appointment, everything healed until there was only a pinprick of a hole left. This was incredibly exciting because it meant that I did not need another surgery to close the hole. I had to continue wearing the boot while this minute hole healed because fluid along the tendon kept coming out of that hole and kept it open. Every time I moved my ankle, it would move along the tendon. The hole was directly over the tendon, which is what compounded the difficulty of healing everything. I did not, however, need surgery, and I was able to cancel it.

About one week after the date my surgery was scheduled, I went in for a CT scan to see if the fractures had healed. We hoped and prayed that they had because, in the past, wearing the boot had not healed the fractures, and that is why it had to be operated on in the first place, which then started this entire infection disaster. I was told that we did not want to check on the fracture until the hole in my ankle had healed or was incredibly close to healing, because no one could do anything about the fracture while there was an open hole. Plus, the first treatment option would be wearing a boot, which I was already doing to help keep my ankle from moving and bending, which kept the hole open. I was nervous about this CT scan, however, because if there was still a fracture or multiple fractures, we would likely need to pursue the next and only other treatment option in my case, which would be surgery. Again, this is how the whole infection situation started, and we wanted to avoid any additional surgeries.

Shortly after I had the CT scan, the results were released to me via the patient portal, and it was determined that the fractures had healed and were no longer present. This news was met with a large sigh of relief, and after meeting with the plastic surgeon, I was able to FINALLY ditch the boot and walk with two shoes of the same style, color, and size, which was wonderful. I wish that I could say things went back to normal, but the scar from the gaping hole in my ankle/foot left me with a lot of nerve pain. Remember, I already had nerve-related issues on the right side of my body from my chronic back pain, so there are already times when I could barely feel large parts of my right foot. In addition, I was still experiencing some pain and swelling, which I was told could last up to a year after the initial injury. Finally, the scar and surrounding skin on my foot and ankle are extremely stretched, and I can feel it pulling, so I may need to do some deep tissue massaging and skin manipulation in the future. However, I am extremely grateful that everything in the ankle/foot wound closed and that it did not require further surgeries to do so.

You may think that this is the end of the issues with my ankles and feet, but after being out of the boot for one month or so, I started experiencing a significant amount of pain and swelling in my left foot, which was the opposite side of the broken ankle. I went to Urgent Care and learned that I had fractured two bones in my foot. Again, I had no idea how or why it happened. So, I was put back into a boot, but this time it was on the left side. I was monitored closely by the podiatry department, and about 6-8 weeks after I found out about the two initial fractures in my foot, I found out that I had fractured ANOTHER bone next to the initial two bones that had fractured. I am not sure how I managed to do this, but somehow I fractured another bone while in the boot. It took months to heal from these three fractures, but eventually, I was able to start wearing shoes of the same size again.

Again, I am not sure how I injured any of the bones in my foot or my ankle, but the podiatrist indicated that my bones looked a bit thin in my feet and ankles. They think that this could possibly be from the chemotherapy drugs that I was given for the neuroblastoma. In addition, another reason why they may have so easily broken and then taken so long to heal is because of the daily steroids that I need to take for the adrenal insufficiency disease. However, I need to take the steroids into account for not producing any cortisol naturally. Overall, we are not quite sure why everything happened at one time and things were so severe, but I hope that the pain and swelling will continue to subside and that I will not have any other fractures in my feet or ankles.

The Spoon Theory

The effects of chronic pain and chronic medical conditions can be difficult to understand, even when you are the one experiencing the effects. Thus, it can be extremely difficult for loved ones, friends, and others to understand, too. The best example that explains the effects of chronic pain and chronic illness, and what it feels like, is the "spoon theory," created by Christine Miserandino. I was introduced to this explanation by a friend only a few short years ago, and it felt like a light turned on because I finally had a complete, detailed and succinct way to explain the effects of my chronic pain, my adrenal insufficiency disease, and the plethora of other medical conditions that affect my daily life.

To explain the "spoon theory," Christine, who had been meeting a friend at a restaurant, gathered a handful of spoons. She explained that each spoon represented a finite unit of energy, and healthy people have an unlimited number of spoons to get through each day. People with chronic illnesses, however, may have a total of 12 spoons per day, but they may need to ration these spoons and use them differently to make it through the day. For example, on a high-pain day, it may take me three spoons to get up and get ready for the day, three spoons to make and eat lunch, and three spoons to do some work. If I have 12 spoons of energy to make it through each day, I only have three spoons of energy left to make it through the rest of my day. So, there are days when I do not have the spoons or energy left to meet socially with family or friends. I often have a difficult time making it through an entire day without resting at some point. However, on a good pain day, it may not take me as many spoons for an activity, leaving me more spoons/energy to do and accomplish other things during my day. The Washington Post has an article with some excellent illustrations that explain the "spoon theory." The article urges others to be mindful of people with chronic conditions who have fewer spoons to make it through the day. The author's friends check on her and can tell when she has fewer spoons and energy each day, and my loved ones, or "Inner Circle," are the same way. "Even though you can't change how many spoons we have left, just knowing you understand can make them last longer."

Conclusion

My medical issues have affected my life differently at various points in time, and even though I have had to make alterations and modifications to my life for some of them, I try not to let them dictate and control my life. At times, it would be quite easy for me to think about all of my medical issues and how they have already impacted my life, and will continue to impact my life in the future. I could wallow over all of the things that I cannot do because of my medical issues, and be depressed about the fact that, although my back pain feels almost unbearable at this point, it will likely just continue to worsen as I get older. And please know, I have those times when I have been incredibly depressed, dealing with my pain and the lack of good pain control. This is accompanied by feelings of being terrified that the pain will worsen, that I will not be able to manage it, and that I could sink into a state of despair, pain, and depression. In my humble opinion, this would be no way to live, and I would rather focus on the fact that I survived childhood cancer; have hope, positivity, and optimism; and fight every day to conquer and deal with my late effects.

So, it may not be a surprise that I wrote this book with some apprehension and trepidation for a few reasons. The purpose of this book is not to complain or gain attention or sympathy for all of the medical issues that I have had or continue to have as a long-term childhood cancer survivor diagnosed in 1980. This has been something that I have feared throughout my life, and is likely why I have not discussed a lot of this before now. It may come as no surprise that this book is very revealing and exposes my life and things that I have never discussed with people or that I have only discussed with my "Inner Circle" of loved ones.

Many of the medical and other experiences written about in this book are extremely personal, and I held much of it in so that no one would know my medical conditions, innermost thoughts, and difficult experiences. However, my philosophy has changed as I have aged and as I have further worked in the nonprofit world. In this time of social media, in which many people reveal the most intimate details of their lives and extremely personal feelings regularly, it can feel unusual for someone to keep things personal and not discuss them. I am a private person, so this is quite new for me; however, I have become a bit more comfortable discussing my medical issues with the neuroblastoma and childhood cancer community because I feel like these are "my people."

We all have childhood cancer in common, and we share some of the same experiences, issues, and feelings, so I feel like we truly understand and relate to each other. They inherently understand me before I say anything because they have either seen it or heard about a friend having it, or they have been through it themselves, either as a patient, survivor, parent/caregiver, or as part of their work with a nonprofit organization. I do not have to explain the very basics of myself like I would need to do with the general public, because this is a community that already knows. My relationships in the childhood cancer community are truly with some of the best people that I know, and they genuinely care about me, keep tabs on me, and remember when I have important things going on so that they can check on me. This has been a wonderful community for me to start sharing more of myself and ease into the revealing nature of an entire book. Furthermore, I have a strong desire to help past, present, and future childhood cancer patients, survivors, and their families, as well as bring awareness, education, and funding to childhood cancer and childhood cancer survivors. My philosophy with nonprofit work has always been that if I can do something to help, then I need to do it. I am now expanding this philosophy to my book by trying to bring attention to important childhood cancer and survivorship issues.

Additionally, I often write about my chronic pain and sometimes question whether discussing it may come across as complaining. Chronic pain is often misunderstood, and I consider myself fortunate to have an "Inner Circle" of individuals who understand this aspect of my life. However, expressing this to the outside world is more challenging, as I genuinely do not want it to seem like I'm merely listing complaints. Growing up, my parents and I seldom talked about my medical issues unless it was with very close friends or if someone specifically inquired about a related medical condition or my chronic pain, fearing it might be perceived as complaining. My parents were concerned that if I frequently discussed my health, people might shy away from engaging with me. Therefore, I am particularly sensitive about this topic and strive to limit conversations regarding my medical issues. Nevertheless, this book aims to share aspects of my life with you, which necessitates discussing and explaining my medical history, late effects, and pain.

Overall, the purpose of this book is not to focus on my ailments but rather to share my experiences, the things that I have learned, and the mentalities, perspectives, and beliefs that I have learned from my personal experiences and that have helped me get through difficult times and life in general. I am not saying that I am especially wise or that you should copy exactly what I have done in my life. Yet, I do have a unique story that has both forced and allowed me to learn and develop some interesting ideas and coping strategies about life. I am hoping that this book will help someone get through their trials and tribulations, whether they are large or small issues, and encourage them to consider different or new ways of thinking.

The majority of people do not understand what it is like to be a cancer survivor, especially a childhood cancer survivor. There is often the mistaken belief that once cancer treatments have been completed, a person reverts to their former self and will never deal with the repercussions of cancer again. This belief, however, is entirely incorrect, and unless childhood cancer has touched a person in some way, people are unable to understand that childhood cancer treatments are extremely toxic. Late effects and other medical issues plague childhood cancer survivors long after treatment has ended, and these late effects can sometimes be as deadly as the cancer itself. Since many people have never experienced childhood cancer or even a serious medical issue, it can be very difficult for them to understand that childhood cancer can continue long after treatment has ended, and it can be a lonely burden for a child or survivor to carry.

Although I have many aspects to my personality, and there is so much more to me than my cancer and my other medical issues, they do affect my everyday life. Due to a variety of medical issues, I am just not able to get outside of my house and be as social as I would like. People are very busy with their own lives, and it typically never occurs to them to think about a person like me who is in severe pain at all times and has numerous medical conditions that confine her to the couch. To know what that feels like is not usually in someone's thoughts because it is so far removed from their own lives, which is completely understandable. However, sometimes all I can do is think, especially about the people in my life, so it can be difficult for me to understand what the "normal" person deals with daily. To bridge that gap, we have tried to invite family and friends to gather at our home so that I can take part in events. With certain people, this has worked, but other family members and friends have not caught on yet, or they simply have ignored our requests and pleas. However, that does not mean that we will stop trying.

My life has been incredibly enriched in so many ways by what I have learned and experienced. I have deep, meaningful relationships, I have gained a tremendous amount of empathy and sensitivity for people, and I have learned about perspective and developed strong values of hope, positivity, and optimism, even in the most difficult of times, as well as faith, love, kindness, and understanding. Yet, this can be entirely frustrating, hurtful, and REALLY lonely. These difficulties and challenges teach valuable lessons and can help enrich our lives. Yet, I also have to keep telling myself that not everyone is going to care. And that is okay.

Lessons, Principles, and Perspectives

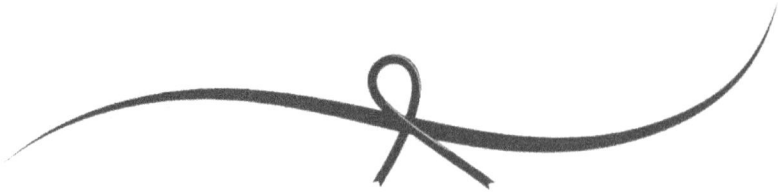

$\mathcal{A}$t any time in my life, if you had asked me what I wanted to do what my ultimate goals were, I would have responded that I wanted to help others and make a meaningful impact in the world. Whether that was through being a doctor, veterinarian, pharmacist, lawyer specializing in healthcare law, or working with a childhood cancer nonprofit, I wanted to explore every avenue. My unique story and experiences with neuroblastoma and the severe, painful late effects from the cancer and its treatments motivated me to use my journey to support and help others.

In 1980, my neuroblastoma diagnosis came at a time when very few children survived any form of cancer. My experimental treatments and the various secondary and late effects I faced, and continue to face, have imparted unique life lessons, principles, and perspectives that hold great significance in my life. These include:

- Hope, optimism, and positivity
- Faith
- A thirst for knowledge
- Humor
- The love and support of my "Inner Circle"
- Having an outlet (for me, that is music)
- Giving back, through my work with various nonprofit organizations

For the patients, survivors, parents/caregivers, and families that read this book, I hope that you can see glimpses of your own story and that these life lessons can help you throughout your own journey with childhood cancer. Additionally, it is essential to understand that while the core of my narrative centers around childhood cancer and survivorship, the lessons and insights within this book can resonate with anyone who has faced, or is currently facing, a challenging situation or experience in life. Even if you haven't experienced childhood cancer or its effects, these insights can still resonate with you and enrich your own journey.

Hope, Optimism, and Positivity

It may seem unusual to discuss the "silver lining" or how to maintain hope, optimism, and positivity during the challenges of childhood cancer, but valuable lessons can emerge from the most difficult situations. This doesn't imply that the experiences weren't difficult, nor does it suggest that you should always focus on positivity or the lessons learned. Instead, it calls for introspection and a cumulative view of the situation.

It is easy to feel angry and let those emotions take control. While it's natural to experience anger at times, it's crucial to step back and reevaluate. Harboring anger and negativity can be detrimental, as it diverts your focus and energy into those feelings. The same applies to consistently feeling sad about your situation. While I'm not implying that you should never feel down about being sick, facing medical challenges, or enduring pain, it's essential to avoid remaining in that mindset.

You need a spark of hope, alongside optimism and positivity, not just to survive but to thrive, achieve your goals, feel good about yourself, assist others, and live life to the fullest. Given the brevity of life, we should strive to embrace each day with purpose.

Many of us experience hardships, but what truly matters is our response to them. You can either allow these difficulties to bring you down, dwell on them, and let them negatively shape your life, or you can choose to transform your perspective. Embrace the opportunity to learn valuable lessons and focus on what you have, as well as how you can help others. One crucial lesson is the importance of optimism and focusing on the positive aspects of life, finding the silver lining in every situation. Whether it's as simple as a kind word, a smile, someone holding the door for you, the unconditional love of a pet, or realizing the immense love and support from your family, friends, and community, there is always something uplifting and optimistic to focus on.

As a child, I often grew weary of hearing my parents repeat the phrase, "The Power of Positive Thinking." This mindset, along with the internationally bestselling book of the same name, was created by Norman Vincent Peale, an American minister, author, and true optimist. He believed that anyone could overcome life's challenges through positivity, optimism, and hope. Peale famously stated, "Change your thoughts and you change your world."

While you cannot alter the reality that challenges will arise, you can work to transform how you think, respond, and cope with them. Even during the toughest days, there is always a silver lining to be discovered, and shifting your perspective can wield tremendous power.

To this day, I strive to live my life in alignment with Peale's beliefs. As you have read, I have many late effects, some of which are quite serious and life-changing. Therefore, maintaining a positive mindset is essential for managing them daily. Overall, the qualities of hope, optimism, and positivity have been instrumental in navigating my medical challenges and other tough situations. Even in the darkest moments, we can discover glimmers of hope and positivity.

While we may strive for control over our emotions, mental health can sometimes make it challenging to maintain a positive or optimistic outlook. It is essential to recognize and embrace the full range of emotions that life brings. After all, if you have not experienced devastation and sadness, how can you truly appreciate the beauty of joy, happiness, and delight? When I find myself feeling depressed, I aim to address it promptly, as the longer I remain in that state, the harder it becomes to overcome. My parents have played a crucial role in my journey, providing a listening ear, offering gentle advice, and prompting me to reflect on my feelings. My dad holds a master's degree in psychology and taught high school psychology, among other subjects. Interestingly, he also served as the guidance counselor and principal at the same high school my brother and I attended. While I had my dad as my guidance counselor in high school, my brother experienced him as the principal (I like to think I had it a bit easier). Throughout our childhood and adolescence, my brother and I engaged in profound discussions about life and mental health with our dad, and his insights and wisdom were truly invaluable.

I used to *never* talk about my cancer, keeping it a closely guarded secret. I didn't want anyone to focus on that aspect of my life. I simply wished to be like every other child my age. The thought of children or adults asking me questions about my condition made me uncomfortable. I had been taught that talking about my medical problems could be perceived as complaining, and very few people wanted to spend time with someone who complained.

Growing up in a small Midwest town with a population of about 1,300, everyone was aware of each other's business. Once someone learned something about a person, it was unlikely to be forgotten. Information often became gossip, shared and discussed at local gathering spots like hair salons, restaurants, bars, churches, and other social venues.

I also had some visual and physical differences that set me apart from my classmates. I was consistently several years behind on growth charts, my Horner's syndrome caused one of my eyes to appear smaller, I would only sweat on one side of my body, I wore various back braces, and I had multiple scars from the numerous surgeries I underwent. These traits could easily become topics of gossip within the town.

Thus, it is ironic and amusing that I have written a book to share with everyone. I realize that many of the "secrets" I have kept so carefully hidden are now being exposed in such a public way. However, I feel somewhat more equipped to share these insights because, over the past few years, I have begun to peel back the layers and open up about my experiences within the neuroblastoma and childhood cancer communities. These communities are incredibly kind and inclusive, where many individuals reach out by sharing their stories, asking questions, discussing feelings, seeking guidance, and essentially learning from one another. People care about each other and just want to help, whether they are a parent or caregiver, a current patient, or a survivor.

Nonprofit organizations focused on neuroblastoma and childhood cancer, along with supportive Facebook groups, have created a nurturing and safe space for me to share personal experiences I have kept hidden for so long. I discovered that my voice holds value, and by reaching out to share my cancer journey or simply offering support and a listening ear to parents, caregivers, patients, and survivors, I could fulfill the childhood dream of helping others and making a meaningful impact.

This realization was transformative and laid the groundwork for my ongoing efforts to fight against neuroblastoma and childhood cancer through education, advocacy, awareness, and fundraising. Since embarking on this mission, I have felt an unprecedented sense of fulfillment. This work provides me with purpose and direction in my life, and I eagerly anticipate continuing it now and in the future.

I have also discovered that I can use my story and experiences with childhood cancer to help others. Although my medical issues require me to rest and prevent me from engaging in a "conventional" job, I remain committed to being productive and feeling valuable. Consequently, I have created a fulfilling life with work that I can accomplish from home, using my laptop while resting on the couch with my therapy cat, Isaac. To support others, I have collaborated with various neuroblastoma, childhood cancer, and cancer-related nonprofit organizations simultaneously. At one point, I worked with as many as ten different organizations at the same time. Additionally, I have participated in public speaking and writing, with a strong desire to expand my efforts in these areas.

With my various medical conditions and chronic pain, I often find myself resting on the couch. However, I make a conscious effort to stay productive and occupied because I believe that if I am going to be in pain regardless, I might as well engage in activities that make me feel valuable and useful. This is a Buddhist proverb that I hold close during tough times: "Pain is inevitable; suffering is optional." We all encounter pain or challenges in life, some more than others. What truly matters is how we respond to that pain or those challenges. You can choose to let it bring you down, dwell in it, and allow it to define your life negatively, or you can harness that pain and those difficulties to cultivate greater determination, gain valuable insights, and concentrate on what you have in life while finding ways to support others. While I experience tough days, just like everyone else, I strive to keep my focus on the positive aspects of my life.

Remember when I was in junior high, wearing my back brace, and a classmate would toss me into the garbage can? Fast forward to my late 30s or early 40s, during a doctor's appointment, when a technician and I began reminiscing about high school and the unkind acts our classmates inflicted upon us. I recounted a few incidents, including the time I was thrown into that garbage can, feeling like a turtle flipped onto its back, utterly helpless. As the bell rang, students hurried through the halls, heading to and from their classes, and they had the chance to walk past me, pointing and laughing as if I were some kind of tourist attraction. Even those I believed would come to my aid disappointed me; they chose to ignore the scene rather than confront our peers who were perpetuating the cruelty.

He inquired whether the "friend" who had wronged me ever expressed remorse later in life, considering we both acknowledged that people often grow and feel regret for their past actions. I was somewhat taken aback by the question, as I had never received an apology for any teasing I experienced, nor had I anticipated one. It can be quite daunting for someone to confront their childhood misdeeds, approach the person they hurt, and offer an apology, especially if they have significantly changed since then. I always believed that such apologies were uncommon, so I informed him that she had not offered one. I also pointed out the irony that she is now a teacher! The technician found it appalling that she had not apologized and mentioned that it would be challenging for him to forgive her, let alone maintain a friendly connection with her on Facebook or in other contexts.

This reflection prompted me to delve deeper into the challenging, teasing, and bullying experiences I faced during my primary and secondary education. (Back when I was in elementary, junior high, and high school, the term "bullying" wasn't commonly used; we simply referred to such behaviors as "mean", "teasing", or other descriptive words that seemed appropriate. I will leave it to you to decide if these actions qualify as bullying, teasing, or something else.) While these experiences were painful and led to many tears, they also taught me resilience. I learned to appear tough and tried not to let my classmates see how much it affected me. Even if my toughness was initially an act, it revealed an inner strength that helped me navigate those difficult times.

I have always been quite a sensitive person, perhaps even more so during my younger years. While I still tend to be more sensitive than most, the emotional and physical teasing I experienced taught me how to navigate difficult situations. Moreover, it revealed to me how I never wanted to behave or communicate, demonstrating how words and actions can profoundly hurt others. These instances of teasing and bullying also deepened my empathy for others, particularly my classmates who faced similar treatment. Although I was often painfully shy at that time, I made an effort to show kindness to all my classmates, even if it was just through a timid smile.

Additionally, I reflected on the technician's comment that he could not move past these actions without an apology. This perspective grants significant power to the bully, as remaining stuck in those experiences could be detrimental to me. We cannot compel others to act as we wish, and I certainly did not need an apology to move forward. I had never considered it this way before. Instead, I choose to view the bullying as experiences that shaped who I am today. Not only have I navigated various medical challenges, but I also endured school while facing some cruel teasing, and I emerged intact. Like many situations, I could choose to see this negatively and allow it to harm me, but I believe that forgiveness can benefit both the wronged and the wrongdoer. This is the perspective I have chosen to adopt. Ultimately, I prefer to focus on what I have gained from being teased and bullied and how it has made me stronger.

When I was diagnosed with neuroblastoma, my life was changed forever. In the past, I hadn't celebrated a "cancerversary," which refers to celebrating the anniversary of a significant event in one's cancer journey, such as the date of diagnosis, the date of a transplant, or the last day of treatment. For me, my cancerversary points to June 6, 1980, the day I received my diagnosis. As a child, I never considered celebrating that day because my family and I were unaware of this notion. However, after engaging with the childhood cancer community and learning about cancerversaries and their significance, I began to acknowledge my own. Having been diagnosed in 1980, I reached 45 years since that pivotal day on June 6, 2025. While my birthday comes a few weeks earlier, I truly believe my cancerversary held an even greater significance than my birthday.

I struggle with the idea of celebrating myself, and I was unsure about how to approach a cancerversary. Therefore, I chose to find a way to honor the many children I was meeting virtually and learning about through their parents. For one of the first cancerversaries I celebrated, I wrote the following tribute to honor the children who were cancer patients in the hospital at that time:

If adults could take life with a little bit more of a childlike perspective, I think that life would be so much more positive, uplifting, and meaningful. We should hope, laugh, live, and love like children, especially like children who are living with and fighting against childhood cancer. If you could spend just one moment with these children, you would see the strength that they have, despite the illness that is ravaging their little bodies and the toxic, horrendous treatments that they must endure to have a chance at living. One might think that being around these little ones could be incredibly heartbreaking, and it most certainly can be, but there is an entirely different side to these children that is absolutely inspirational. First, you can clearly see the courage in each child, and that is a very necessary quality that is needed to fight cancer. They also exude such love and affection, but they also seem to have a blind, unwavering faith that they will get better. Many times, the ill children will buoy the strength and resolve of their parents, which is truly remarkable considering all that they are going through.

One of the ways that we can get through difficult situations is through laughter. Despite being poked, prodded, scanned, and put through more procedures than anyone could possibly count, children with cancer still manage to laugh throughout the day, as well as make everyone around them laugh. And, is anything more beautiful than the sound of children laughing, especially when the average person would expect them to be sad and crying?. These children with cancer continue to amaze me with their strength, sense of humor, bravery, positive beliefs, and their overall sense of hope. Honestly, the average American seems to complain about every little thing, which can get them down and put a negative spin on the day. However, if they could just observe a child fighting cancer and the amazing attitudes that they possess, it might put a little more perspective on their own lives. In fact, I think that it could change their perspectives entirely, and for the better, if they could just observe children who are fighting childhood cancer.

I want my life to mean something and to help people. I believe that my survival serves multiple purposes. Beyond offering hope, I aim for my nonprofit efforts to create a lasting impact. I engage with several childhood cancer organizations in various roles, as I feel a strong responsibility to raise awareness for both childhood cancer patients and survivors through my work.

Additionally, I wish to share my cancer journey, including my experiences with numerous late effects as a survivor, along with my insights and philosophies on life. My goal is for others to learn from my experiences and perhaps derive some benefit from them. I hope my story inspires people to discover ways to cultivate hope, positivity, and optimism in their own lives, even amid despair, challenges, and hardships.

As previously stated, many individuals have faced challenging experiences. You can choose to let these hardships overwhelm you, or you can harness them to pursue an extraordinary and joyful life. I am a childhood cancer survivor who has endured and continues to endure various significant medical challenges that have profoundly affected my life. These medical issues will remain with me for the rest of my life, and they may worsen as I age. Moreover, late effects from childhood cancer can emerge many years or even decades after treatment, which means I could potentially face new medical conditions in the future. Nevertheless, each day I consciously strive to focus on the brighter side and embrace the positive, hopeful elements of every situation.

Hope is incredibly important, and I choose to believe it exists in every circumstance, regardless of how dire the situation may seem. Through my journey, I have discovered that hope, optimism, and positivity are essential for navigating the challenging aspects of life, including recurring serious medical issues, late effects, cancer scares, episodes of anxiety and depression, and more.

As I mentioned earlier, I do experience tough days emotionally, spiritually, and physically. Each of us faces difficult times, and it is important to acknowledge and feel those emotions. However, if I allow myself to dwell in negativity for too long, it becomes challenging to rise above it. Therefore, I strive to extract lessons from these experiences and then move forward.

I believe that facing hardships, weaknesses, and challenges can impart profound wisdom and teach us invaluable lessons. This understanding has truly enriched my life and helped me navigate through tough times. Additionally, I've identified several "building blocks" (methods and activities) that foster hope, optimism, and positivity in my life, and I hope that as I share them, they will encourage you in your journey.

A Thirst for Knowledge

While my numerous medical challenges have significantly influenced my life, they do not define my entire existence. My medical journey has shaped my philosophy and outlook, leading me to realize that a thirst for knowledge is a crucial life principle that fosters hope, optimism, and positivity. Knowledge does not always have to be tied to traditional education. Initially, I pursued a conventional education because it was essential for achieving my career aspirations, which included my childhood dreams of becoming a doctor or veterinarian, and as an adult, a pharmacist or a lawyer focusing on healthcare law or working with a childhood cancer nonprofit organization.

With both of my parents in the field of education, I learned the value of college at a young age. I was quite young when I set my sights on becoming the valedictorian of my high school class. This ambition was inspired by witnessing my babysitter's son achieve that honor, which made my grades a top priority throughout my educational journey, especially in high school. I recognized that I was not a natural "genius," someone who easily excelled academically. Instead, I had to put in a considerable amount of effort to achieve the grades necessary to become the valedictorian of the 1997 Galesville-Ettrick-Trempealeau High School graduating class.

Yet, only a handful of people beyond my immediate family were aware that I aspired to be the valedictorian. Several students were far more intelligent than I, and two in particular were anticipated to receive the honor. Thus, when it was revealed during the latter part of my senior year that I had been named valedictorian, many were taken aback. They had no idea I was even in the running, as I rarely discussed my academic achievements.

In Wisconsin, the valedictorian is awarded free tuition to a state university of their choice. Additionally, I dedicated a significant amount of time during my senior year to applying for various scholarships, which covered my room, food, supplies, and more. I realized how fortunate I was to have my undergraduate education completely funded, graduating in just three and a half years with a Bachelor of Science (BS) degree in political science. During the latter half of that semester, I underwent another major back surgery, using that time to recover, work from home for the legal department of a local medical center, and prepare for law school.

I believe I was destined to be a student and absorb as much knowledge as I could. Initially, when I entered college, I planned to attend for two years and take pre-pharmacy courses, which focused heavily on biology and chemistry. However, I found myself struggling with some of these subjects, particularly organic chemistry and calculus. Rather than continue with courses that I really did not like, I decided to pivot dramatically and switch my major to political science! Interestingly, I made this decision before even taking a political science class. Fortunately, my intuition about enjoying this field proved correct, and I graduated with a perfect 4.0 in my major.

After earning my BS in political science, I decided to pursue a graduate degree through law school. However, law school imparted a significant lesson. Following a semester at a law school in St. Louis, Missouri, I realized that this was not the right career path for me. That single semester proved to be a considerable financial burden, especially since I had relocated my entire life to St. Louis for what I expected would be at least three years of study. Alongside the expense and upheaval, I was heartbroken, feeling adrift without a clear sense of what career or further education I should pursue.

This period was profoundly challenging, as I grappled with feelings of failure and confusion. On the bright side, I was able to return home and spend time every day with my boyfriend, who would later become my husband. I also learned that it is perfectly acceptable to reconsider one's choices and acknowledge that a pursued path may not be the right fit. More importantly, had I been able to foresee the future, I would have recognized that my health issues were beginning to escalate, significantly affecting my life and preventing me from becoming a practicing lawyer. The crucial lesson I took away from this experience is that God is indeed in control of my life. Although it was incredibly tough to accept that law school was not meant for me and that I needed to seek a new career direction, He guided me through that difficult time. Ultimately, I went on to pursue and earn a more versatile Master of Business Administration (MBA) degree, also from the University of Wisconsin-La Crosse.

When I realized that pursuing the professional career I had envisioned was no longer possible, I began to question how I could still make a meaningful impact in people's lives. I longed to feel productive, worthwhile, and valuable. After enduring years of painful injuries, major surgeries, and chronic severe back pain caused by scoliosis and multiple fusion surgeries of my spine, along with years of medication that left me feeling like a zombie, my aspirations seemed increasingly out of reach.

As the medication was reduced, I gradually began to rediscover myself. I became involved with nonprofits focused on neuroblastoma and childhood cancer, and I realized I could create a positive impact by sharing my story. Although I have not utilized my degrees in a traditional professional capacity, I genuinely believe they have equipped me for my fight against childhood cancer. Moreover, I continue to learn and grow in my roles within the childhood cancer community, and this ongoing education is something I truly cherish.

Additionally, in March 2021, I had the opportunity to share my story and nonprofit work in an interview with Mark Levine on the *Help and Hope Happen Here* podcast. Mark is an incredible individual who had organized various fundraising events for childhood cancer, but when the pandemic struck, all his plans were abruptly interrupted. He contemplated how he could continue to support the childhood cancer community, leading to the creation of his podcast, which remains active today. Mark and I connected immediately and have maintained regular email communication, meeting in person several times at CureFest for Childhood Cancer in Washington, D.C. During our discussions, we talked about my book, and he made it his personal mission to find a publisher for it. He succeeded in finding the perfect match!

Mark had also interviewed Dana-Susan Crews for his podcast. From the age of seven, when her brother was diagnosed with cancer, Dana-Sue became deeply involved in the world of childhood cancer, dedicating her life to combat it through various means. One significant avenue has been the Bell Asteri Publishing Company, which focuses exclusively on publishing books about childhood cancer, aiming to enhance "the lives of the children in the cancer community through the art of storytelling." Bell Asteri stands out among publishing companies, and Dana-Sue is a truly wonderful, kind, and caring individual. We are also both members of the Gold Together Advisory Council (more on this later), and we have met several times in person. She truly has become a genuine friend. Dana-Sue is incredibly generous, often covering various expenses for her authors, and she donates proceeds from her books to pediatric cancer research, advocacy, and other initiatives.

Throughout my journey of completing my book, Dana-Sue has been patient and understanding, especially as I worked on two survivorship programs for the Coalition Against Childhood Cancer (CAC2). These programs demanded significant time and delayed my book's completion, yet Dana-Sue offered only support and empathy as a friend, colleague, and exceptional publisher/editor.

In 2022, I was able to meet both Mark and Dana-Sue in person for the first time and express my gratitude for everything they had done for me. It was a surreal experience, and I had someone capture a photo of the three of us because, without either of them, I would not have been able to finish my book and hold a published copy in my hands. Fortunately, Dana-Sue, Mark, and I reunited at CureFest in both 2023 and 2024, spending precious moments together. We are also expected to spend time together at CureFest 2025, too. However, time is always limited at conferences, as I often assist multiple nonprofits while attending. Therefore, it's essential to cherish our time together and make the most of it.

Writing my book has probably been the most significant learning experience I have ever had. I had to delve deep into both painful and joyful memories to gain a better understanding of myself. I feel as though my self-discovery is ongoing, and I aspire to continue this journey throughout my life. Additionally, I conducted extensive research on medical topics, ensuring that I communicated this information clearly and understandably for my readers. This process led me to explore not only my own medical experiences but also the stories and insights of others. I am grateful to Mark, Dana-Sue, and Bell Asteri Publishing for their support in helping me complete my book, which has truly been a remarkable learning journey.

Faith

I grew up with a strong sense of faith and religion. We were ELCA (Evangelical Lutheran Church in America) Lutherans, which is a very liberal denomination and has really suited me and my beliefs throughout my life. As a child, my family went to church every week at Zion Lutheran Church in Galesville, Wisconsin. It was there where my brother and I attended Sunday School from the age of three or four to throughout high school, which was as long as it extended. I even played the piano for church services and sang with the choir, but I also played the oboe.

As a result of my background, I have continued to engage with my church community in various ways. We became members of Good Shepherd Lutheran Church in La Crosse around 2018, where I sing soprano in the Sanctuary Choir and play the oboe in the instrumental ensemble, Sounds of Praise. (It's worth mentioning that I had to take a few breaks from attending church during COVID, as I was navigating my "ankle saga" and recovering from multiple surgeries. However, I have enjoyed attending services online from home.) Additionally, I have developed a close friendship with Pastor Harald Bringsjord, our pastor at Good Shepherd Lutheran Church, and we have had countless conversations covering a wide range of topics.

During Lent, church members are invited to share messages during the Wednesday services, and I was honored to be invited to deliver one of these messages in 2019. I was the first to speak that year, coinciding with the first day of Lent, which was also Ash Wednesday. The Gospel beautifully aligned with my personal story, and I believe it is important to share it here, as it illustrates my faith and how it supports me through my medical challenges.

In Paul's second letter to the Corinthians, Chapter 12, verses 9-10, he shares a powerful message: "My grace is sufficient for you, for power is made perfect in weakness." Paul states that he will gladly boast of his weaknesses, as it allows the power of Christ to reside within him. Consequently, he finds contentment in weaknesses, insults, hardships, persecutions, and calamities for the sake of Christ; for it is in his weakness that he discovers strength.

I have been told that I possess a deep understanding of suffering, having experienced it from a young age, much like Paul did. The purpose of sharing my story is not to complain about my numerous medical issues, seek sympathy, or earn praise. Rather, I aim to recount some of the hardships I've faced and illustrate how these challenging experiences, often perceived as weaknesses, have shaped me into a stronger individual.

In the second part of this book, you read about various hardships and weaknesses I've encountered and will continue to face throughout my life. However, it is essential to recognize that everyone experiences difficulties in life. Further, as we learned from Paul, his journey was far from perfect, filled with struggles, challenges, and weaknesses.

When examining the Greek origin of the word "weakness," three distinct definitions emerge:

- Suffering from a debilitating illness or being unwell
- Facing personal incapacity or limitations
- Experiencing a lack of material necessities, being in need

With these definitions, the exact nature of Paul's weakness remains unclear, and we cannot pinpoint which one he encountered. However, Paul speaks of being content with his weaknesses. While I may not label myself as "content," I have accepted my medical challenges and strive to make the best of my situation. Navigating this can be a daily struggle, and some may question why I am not angry with God regarding my cancer diagnosis and its aftermath. It's important to note that although childhood cancer occurs during youth, its effects can resonate throughout a lifetime.

We may never fully grasp why certain events occur in our lives or why we endure suffering. Understanding God's intentions can feel like an impossible endeavor. We must remind ourselves that God does not aim to punish us. God was not punishing me when I got sick, especially as an innocent infant born with a tumor. The one truth we can hold onto is that God loves us. I know He has been by my side through every challenge, providing the strength needed to navigate years of difficulties and medical trials. Much like Paul, I have come to recognize God's strength through my struggles and weaknesses. In moments of weakness, pain, or illness, I feel His strength, which, in turn, empowers me.

For several years, I had the privilege of conversing weekly with my former pastor, Arnold Flater. He was the church pastor during my high school years, and his son, Adam, graduated alongside me. Adam and I were close friends, sharing many interests and participating in various musical ensembles together. Pastor Flater and I discussed numerous topics affecting my life, as well as broader issues, including spirituality and religious matters, and studying various Bible books together. I shared my frustrations about people not understanding or acknowledging my medical challenges, particularly when it involved close family or friends. He provided an insightful perspective on this, explaining that some individuals struggle to confront difficult realities. He has counseled terminal brain cancer patients in their nineties who still cling to the hope of living far into the future, simply because they find it hard to accept tough news.

I know individuals close to me who find it difficult to discuss any negative aspects of life. They prefer to exist in a "happy bubble" and resist anything that might disrupt it. To me, this mindset seems rather sad, as we cannot truly grow and learn without facing challenges and hardships. Just consider how much more you appreciate life's value after experiencing illness or other significant obstacles. Such experiences transform us in countless ways; while they are undeniably tough, the wisdom gained is priceless.

My life has been profoundly enriched by the lessons I've learned and the experiences I've faced. I have developed deep, meaningful relationships, cultivated a strong sense of empathy and sensitivity towards others, and endeavored to embrace values of hope, positivity, and optimism, alongside faith, love, and kindness during the most challenging times.

However, the cornerstone of it all is my faith, especially during days when being strong feels nearly impossible. Faith and religious beliefs can provide a sense of strength, while believing in and praying to a higher power brings peace and comfort. One of my favorite Bible verses that encapsulates this message is from the book of Psalms, Chapter 138, verse 3: "As soon as I pray, You answer me; You encourage me by giving me strength." In tough moments, this verse resonates with me, as I recognize that despite the trials I have endured, God is consistently by my side, guiding me through my struggles.

It is easy to maintain faith when everything is going smoothly, but it is crucial to remember that God remains present, especially during times of hardship and vulnerability. He forgives our sins, and we must also forgive ourselves when our faith falters or when we lose our way amidst difficulties. In moments of weakness, He has made me strong, just as Paul reminds us in his teachings.

Jason Micheli, a United Methodist pastor, authored the book *Cancer is Funny: Keeping Faith in Stage-Serious Chemo*. He faced a diagnosis of Mantle Cell Lymphoma, a rare type of cancer that necessitated intense chemotherapy sessions. Despite being a member of the clergy, Micheli candidly acknowledged that his faith wavered during treatment. His book contains reflections and sentiments that may not align with typical expectations of a clergy member. Yet, he gained profound insights during this challenging period, and he articulated that both in moments of joy and suffering, we can sense God's presence.

Amidst the pain and brutality of cancer and its treatments, Pastor Micheli writes: "Tears, and the suffering that provokes them, can in fact bring us closer to God by leaving us no other options but turning to God. But tears and suffering cannot fetter us to God. Only joy can bind us fully to the God who is the most infallible joy. Cancer is funny, then, because suffering occasioned by cancer draws you nearer to God, and the closer you get to God, the louder laughter becomes... I believe laughter is still the best medicine, but even more so, I've come to believe laughter is the surest sign you're not alone, because joy is the most unmistakable indication of God's presence."

Once Pastor Micheli completed his grueling chemotherapy treatments, he underwent testing and discovered that his cancer was in remission; however, this type of cancer could recur at any moment. Rather than dwell on this uncertainty, he chose to create a "bucket list" filled with enjoyable activities for himself, his wife, and their two sons. One of his first decisions was to get a faith-based tattoo symbolizing his cancer journey and treatment. Pastor Micheli shared with the tattoo artist his learnings from his cancer experience, offering a perspective on suffering and how God supports us through it. He draws a parallel between his struggles during treatment and Jesus' sacrifice on the cross: "In Jesus, God takes all those experiences and emotions of ours into himself... God doesn't cause our pain and suffering. God doesn't shun us because of our shortcomings. God makes them his own. That's how we know we're not alone, because God makes all our junk his own."

God gave us an incredible gift of grace when Jesus died on the cross.

This concept is beautifully illustrated in the 51st Psalm, when David seeks forgiveness and confesses his desire for a "clean heart" from God. Grace is defined as "the free and unmerited favor of love of God, as manifested in the salvation of sinners and the bestowal of blessings." By the grace of God, I overcame childhood cancer in the early 80s, navigated various health challenges, and discovered fulfilling work and purpose, all thanks to divine grace and a deep sense of faith. Ligonier Ministries emphasizes the relationship between grace and the Christian life with this quote: "Christian life is a matter of grace. Grace initiates our salvation, it sustains our salvation, and it will complete our salvation."

Turning to Paul's second letter to the Corinthians, he appeals to the Lord, who reassures him: "My grace is sufficient for you, for power is made perfect in weakness." We all have our vulnerabilities. I certainly have my share. Paul continues, "So, I will boast all the more gladly of my weaknesses, insults, hardships, persecutions, and calamities for the sake of Christ..." Our challenging experiences can either break us or build us up, but with Christ and faith, these trials can impart valuable lessons and empower us to achieve great things. As Paul expresses and I resonate with, "for whenever I am weak, then I am strong." Through our faith and the grace of God, we can all find strength.

Strength can often be depicted using the tiniest of things. During one of my many visits to the doctor, I decided to explore the hospital gift shop for potential gift ideas. While browsing, I stumbled upon a table featuring jewelry, and I noticed some necklaces adorned with a tiny mustard seed at the center charm. Although I had heard various lessons about the mustard seed in Sunday school and during church services, I realized I needed to refresh my memory.

In my research, I discovered three relevant parables, or teachings, that Jesus used in the Bible to reference the mustard seed, which Jesus used to convey his teachings. The mustard seed is mentioned in multiple gospels, and in each of the following verses, it symbolizes the kingdom of heaven and serves as a metaphor for faith. One of the most well-known parables about the mustard seed is found in Matthew 13:31-32, which states: "The kingdom of heaven is like a mustard seed, which a man took and planted in his field. Though it is the smallest of all seeds, yet when it grows, it is the largest of garden plants and becomes a tree, so that the birds of the air come and perch in its branches."

For biologists and purists, this verse may raise some concerns, as the mustard seed is not actually the smallest in existence. That title belongs to a type of orchid seed, which is comparable to dust. Additionally, mustard seeds typically grow into bushes rather than trees, although they can reach impressive heights of 10 feet or more. Thus, it's clear that the mustard seed is neither the "smallest of all seeds" nor does it develop into a tree. However, the significance of using the mustard seed is to convey a particular lesson or parable.

Moreover, during that time and in that region of the world, the mustard seed was familiar to the audience Jesus addressed, making it a fitting example. It's possible that, at that time, it was the smallest seed they were aware of, and its resemblance to a tree as it grew made it a relatable comparison to the largest of the other garden plants.

In addition to the initial parable, I came across two other passages where the disciples approached Jesus with challenges, and He employed the mustard seed to illustrate solutions. In Matthew 17:20, Jesus explained to His disciples why they were unable to cast out a demon afflicting a young boy who was experiencing seizures. He responded, "Because you have so little faith. Truly I tell you, if you have faith as small as a mustard seed, you can say to this mountain, 'Move from here to there,' and it will move. Nothing will be impossible for you."

Moreover, Luke 17:1-11 features Jesus discussing the mustard seed while addressing the challenges of forgiveness. Here are excerpts from verses 3-6: "So watch yourselves. If your brother or sister sins against you rebuke them; and if they repent, forgive them. The apostles then said to the Lord, 'Increase our faith.' He replied, 'If you have faith as small as a mustard seed, you can say to this mulberry tree, 'Be uprooted and planted in the sea, and it will obey you.'"

The mustard seed serves as a metaphor for faith, which embodies a strong feeling or belief in something. As a Christian, I interpret faith as a deep belief in God. However, faith can take many forms, and the mustard seed analogy effectively illustrates a variety of faith interpretations.

A mustard seed is incredibly tiny, and faith can start with the belief in something as small as a tiny seed. Just like a seed, however, these feelings can slowly grow and become a much bigger part of your life. As my faith has grown, it has become pervasive throughout my entire life. When Jesus talks about moving a mountain or moving the mulberry bush, he is not talking about the literal act of doing these actions. Instead, an article on MyRedeemer.org, "The Parable of the Mustard Seed and Faith," discusses that the goal of "moving" these objects is about "taking away the fearful thoughts so that the circumstances are no longer something to dread. Circumstances will no longer control your life because you will trust God to do what is good for you, and for those around you." In other words, the more that your faith grows from that tiny seed, the better your life will be because you are taking things that are beyond your control and that can cause a lot of worry and stress, and you are simply giving them over to God and trusting that he will handle the situation and do what is best for you.

The reason why I gravitated toward this jewelry and Jesus' teachings about the mustard seed is that I know that faith, but also hope, optimism, and positivity, can start with something as small as a mustard seed. These seeds can grow into a large tree with branches, which provide a home and shelter to birds. The "branches" of faith, as well as hope, optimism, and positivity, have the possibility of reaching many, many people in your life, as well as other people that you may never even know have been reached. The amazing thing is that each person that you affect with your faith and positive attitude can create their own "trees" from their mustard seeds, which, in turn, have the capacity to reach many other people that you may never even meet.

I feel the same way about neuroblastoma and pediatric cancer awareness, research, and funding. It all begins with a small seed of an idea, which can blossom into a mighty tree, reaching many individuals who can support the cause of childhood cancer. This growth not only helps raise awareness but also connects with countless childhood cancer patients and survivors. The more we invest in research and develop new treatments and medications, the greater the chance we have of curing pediatric cancer and reducing the likelihood of severe late effects.

Sadly, many people lack an understanding of childhood cancer survivorship, and the challenges faced by survivors often remain unknown. While this is entirely understandable, it can feel isolating and painful, as those who haven't experienced similar circumstances may struggle to grasp the full impact of surviving childhood cancer and the medical complications that can arise. It is my responsibility to convey this reality to others, but I also remind myself that not everyone will take the time to learn about childhood cancer survivorship. Although this reality can be disheartening, it drives me to work even harder. As I pursue my efforts in this field, I must hold onto a steadfast belief that most people will come to care about the experiences of childhood cancer patients and survivors.

Similarly, Jesus encouraged us to cultivate a "childlike faith," urging us to trust in God and His teachings as children do. Children embody innocence and purity, often radiating joy even in the face of challenges, such as those highlighted by Erma Bombeck in her book, *I Want to Grow*

Hair, I Want to Grow Up, I Want to Go to Boise. Children believe without question. Merriam-Webster defines faith, in a religious context, as the "belief, trust in, and loyalty to God...a firm belief in something for which there is no proof." We should embrace the principles of Christianity, or whatever faith we practice, with unwavering belief, striving to maintain an innocent, unquestioning faith without seeking further evidence or examples. Moreover, children exemplify trust and loyalty, and we should mirror this in our religious convictions.

Christianity is often complex, with concepts that can be challenging to grasp. Furthermore, there is no concrete proof that our beliefs are accurate or will manifest as we expect. Yet, children embrace faith without requiring such validation. Many adults struggle with this simplicity, as we tend to overanalyze, judge, and question, often deeming certain beliefs unrealistic. However, children approach the world with trust, understanding, purity, and innocence, believing readily in what they are told. Jesus taught that having faith like children would grant us access to the kingdom of heaven.

Recognizing the perspectives of children is vital, not only in relation to faith and beliefs but also in everyday life. If adults could adopt a childlike viewpoint, life would undoubtedly become more positive and meaningful.

Not only should we hope, laugh, live, love, and have faith like children, but especially like children who are living with childhood cancer. If you spend just a little time with an ill child, you will see the strength and tenacity that they have, despite the illness that is ravaging their little bodies, and the toxic, horrific treatments that they must endure to treat their cancers and give them a chance at survival. You would think that being around these little ones would be so sad and depressing, but you can see the courage in each child. They also exude such love, affection, and typically a blind faith that they will get better at some point in the future. Many times, the ill child will buoy their parents' strength and resolve, which is incredible considering all that they are going through.

Laughter is the Best Medicine

One remarkable way to navigate through tough times is by embracing laughter. Even when faced with countless medical procedures—being poked, prodded, and scanned—a child battling cancer can still find joy and make others laugh. There's nothing more heartwarming and beautiful than the genuine sound of a child's laughter, especially in moments when one might expect tears. Children with cancer never cease to amaze me with their resilience, courage, positive outlook, and humor. Often, they provide strength not just to their parents and family, but also to the broader community. In contrast, many people seem to dwell on trivial complaints, allowing negativity to seep into their lives. If they could witness the spirit and attitude of a typical childhood cancer patient, I believe it would profoundly shift their perspective for the better.

Injecting laughter into my life has always served as a fantastic coping mechanism, offering a joyful way to infuse hope, optimism, and positivity. I genuinely love to laugh, even when it causes discomfort in my chronic pain areas. The adage, "Laughter is the best medicine," holds true, as it brings both physical and emotional benefits to the body.

Laughter serves as an effective tool for stress relief. Research conducted by the Mayo Clinic has revealed numerous short-term and long-term advantages. Among the short-term benefits, laughter triggers physical changes within the body, stimulating various organs. For instance, it enhances the intake of oxygen-rich air and boosts the release of endorphins, our body's natural feel-good chemicals, contributing to an overall sense of well-being and providing temporary pain relief. Additionally, laughter helps alleviate stress, lowers the resting heart rate and blood pressure, stimulates circulation, relaxes muscles, eases tension, and diminishes some physical symptoms associated with stress.

On the other hand, laughter has some wonderful long-term benefits. It can help improve and boost your immune system and fight stress and illnesses. In turn, laughter may ease pain by causing the body to produce natural painkillers. Laughter also relaxes the entire body, and it relieves physical tension and stress for up to 45 minutes. It can strengthen resilience and increase personal satisfaction, making it easier to cope with difficult situations and better connect with others. Finally, in the long term, laughter improves your mood and helps lessen stress, anxiety, and depression, making you feel happier and improving your self-esteem.

Overall, laughter unites people and can strengthen their relationships. Mayo Clinic found that sharing laughter keeps relationships fresh and exciting and can add joy, vitality, and resilience. Furthermore, humor can heal resentments, disagreements, and hurt, and unite people during difficult times. Laughter can also attract others to us, enhance teamwork, help defuse conflict, and promote group bonding.

Laughter also helps your physical health because it relaxes your body, relieves tension and stress, boosts the immune system, triggers the release of endorphins, protects the heart by improving the function of blood vessels and increasing blood flow, burns calories, lessens anger, and can help you live longer. Furthermore, laughter has some mental health benefits, including that it: adds joy to our lives; eases anxiety, tension, and stress; improves mood; and strengthens resilience. Laughter helps stop distressing emotions, it helps you relax and recharge, drawing you closer to others, and it can help you shift perspectives, which is so important for improving your mental health and focusing on hope, optimism, and positivity.

In the book, *Laughter is the Best Medicine*, the author explains that: "Laughter strengthens your immune system, boosts mood, decreases pain, and protects you from the damaging effects of stress... Humor lightens your burdens, inspires hope, connects you to others, and keeps you grounded, focused, and alert. It also helps you release anger and forgive sooner." Finally, it also simply feels good to laugh. Laughter can bring about joy and happiness, and it is fun, free, and easy to do.

Inner Circle

A vital element that has helped me navigate challenging times in my life is the love and support of my "Inner Circle." This group includes my husband, my family (my parents and my brother), the amazing cats I have owned, and some close friends. I am truly blessed to have a fantastic support system, both physically and emotionally, and I am grateful for their unconditional love, assistance, and encouragement. These are the individuals who know everything about me, including the complexities of my medical conditions and the daily struggles I face. They have been instrumental in helping me through tough moments, whether related to health or life in general, and they are the ones with whom I share my joys and victories, loving me no matter what challenges arise.

Growing up, my parents instilled in me the importance of not complaining to others, as many people are not interested in hearing about your troubles, especially regarding medical issues. They taught me that excessive complaining can lead others to avoid spending time with you. I have firsthand experience of this, as I had a high school classmate who frequently voiced her grievances, and eventually, people began to steer clear of her. I never wanted to be perceived that way, so I generally refrain from discussing my medical issues with anyone outside my Inner Circle. They are the ones who listen when I express my pain or when I feel utterly exhausted and depleted of cortisol. Yet, I cannot possibly burden them with every detail of what I am going through all at once.

At times, I have felt very alone and lonely, and people rarely know how much I hurt or how awful I feel because I do not vocalize it. So yes, it is my fault for feeling this way because I do not share everything that I am thinking or feeling. I do not want to be seen as complaining, and I want to protect my loved ones and not burden them with everything. Yet, my "Inner Circle" consists of those I talk to about difficulties with my medical issues, and I truly value, love, and respect them immensely.

Troy:

I have been extremely blessed to find the most loving, caring, wonderful husband. Troy and I started dating in 2001 and got married in 2004, so we have been together for quite some time. He really does take great care of me, and we greatly love and support each other. When we started dating, I was recovering from a major back surgery. At that time, Troy did not have any experience with medical issues or caregiving, but he was introduced to it rather quickly! We went from Troy almost fainting at the first surgery that he experienced with me before we were even married, to being my primary caregiver and cleaning surgical sites.

You know how they say you often meet someone when you least expect it? That was certainly the case for me with Troy. During my undergraduate studies at the University of Wisconsin-La Crosse, I took oboe lessons and performed in the UW-L Orchestra. Many of my close friends at that time were from the orchestra, a pursuit I engaged in purely for enjoyment. In May 2000, the UW-L Orchestra was scheduled for a European tour, performing and sightseeing in the Czech Republic, Poland, Hungary, and Austria.

However, I had already made plans with friends years prior for a spring break trip to Cancun before the orchestra's European tour was announced. After paying for that trip and enjoying it, I felt it was neither fair to ask for additional funds, nor did I have the means to go without doing so. I was prepared to skip the European trip, but the orchestra needed an oboe player. Luckily, I received a scholarship from the orchestra, and my parents generously contributed the remaining cost of the trip as a 21st birthday gift. That journey was incredibly significant in my life, and I cannot imagine my growth and evolution without it! Additionally, I grew closer to several orchestra members, including Amanda, a clarinetist.

Now, how does this connect to Troy? Well, Amanda worked at Menards, a store in the Midwest that sells construction materials, similar to Home Depot and Lowe's. She was a cashier there, and her direct manager was Troy Olson. Having started at Menards just before turning 16, Troy worked his way up through the ranks. He formed friendships with Amanda and other colleagues, although he made an effort to keep his personal relationships separate from his work life.

In 2001, both Troy and Amanda found themselves single on Valentine's Day. Rather than wallowing in self-pity or spending the evening alone, Troy decided to prepare dinner for Amanda at her place, but just as friends. Amanda was aware that I was also without a boyfriend at that time and had recently undergone major back surgery at the end of December, so I was still recovering. She kindly invited me to join them for dinner, but I hesitated at first, not wanting to feel like a third wheel. However, she reassured me that it was a "just friends" gathering and promised an abundance of food, so I agreed. Thus, my "first date" with Troy also included my friend Amanda, and it occurred on Valentine's Day during my recovery from a major back surgery. I never expected to meet a boyfriend, let alone the love of my life, in such a situation.

I was utterly charmed by Troy and everything he did for Valentine's Day. He prepared fettuccine Alfredo with shrimp and brought flowers to decorate the table and share with us. He even picked up a jazz CD to provide the perfect background music (remember, this was 2001, and

CDs were the way to enjoy music). Not to mention, he was quite handsome, and I found our conversations that night truly engaging. Valentine's Day fell on a Wednesday that year, and Amanda planned to host a party at her place on Friday or Saturday. Both Troy and I had separately confided our interest in each other to Amanda, and at her party, we spent the entire night on the couch together, engrossed in conversation. Although there were many guests present, it felt as if we were the only two people in the room. Our connection deepened, and we exchanged phone numbers that evening. From that moment on, we have been in touch nearly every day of our lives!

We made our relationship official at the beginning of March, and it felt remarkably different from any previous relationships I had experienced. For instance, Troy actually followed through on his promises. He called me when he said he would. More significantly, despite being two years younger than I, he was the most mature man I had ever dated. However, we began our relationship at a challenging time. In August 2001, just five months after we started dating. I was enrolled in law school at St. Louis University, which boasted the top healthcare law program in the country at the time. I feared that the best relationship of my life might not last, as long-distance relationships often struggle, and I was committed to being in St. Louis for at least three years. We spoke on the phone every day and made an effort to see each other twice a month, once when I traveled home and once when Troy drove down to visit me. Remember, this was in 2001 when the Internet, video telephone calls, and other technology did not exist. We simply had our cell phones for communication.

During the first semester, we made the most of our situation and truly got to know each other. However, I soon realized that neither law school nor St. Louis was the right fit for me. I decided to return home and enroll in the University of Wisconsin-La Crosse's Master of Business

Administration (MBA) program. The greatest advantage was that Troy and I could see each other every day.

Troy and his family had limited experience with hospitals, clinics, and medical issues, and as I mentioned earlier, he met me right after I had major back surgery. Throughout the time we were dating, I underwent several surgeries and medical procedures, with my parents serving as my primary caregivers. We wanted to gently introduce Troy to the process without overwhelming him, as we aimed to prepare him for the future when we would live together and he would take on the role of my primary caregiver. I still cannot believe how far Troy has come; he transitioned from feeling queasy at the thought of a wound or surgical site to diligently cleaning that site multiple times a day.

Troy proposed to me on my golden birthday, May 24, 2003. This is also the day that his sister, Anna, graduated from high school. He had cleared it with her to make sure she was okay with the proposal on this date. Plus, she had her graduation party on May 25, so we could focus on Anna on that date. Originally, Troy was going to propose to me at the top of a Ferris wheel; however, Troy is slightly afraid of heights, and he kept having a vision of dropping the ring. So, he proposed to me privately, and it was wonderful.

As a childhood cancer survivor, however, even a proposal needs additional education and action. Troy and I dated for more than three years, so my parents were able to slowly have conversations with him about my medical issues. The fact that we did not know if I could have biological children was a topic of conversation, but Troy did not seem to mind. Additionally, when Troy asked my parents if he could marry me, they gave their blessing, but they also made sure to let him know that he would always need to have health insurance for me because one health issue could bankrupt us. For example, just one of my back surgeries was a quarter of a million dollars, and by my 46th birthday, I had already had 52 surgeries, so health insurance was critical. Troy listened to each concern and agreed to everything, thus securing my parents' blessing to ask me to marry him on my golden birthday.

We tied the knot on a stunning spring day, April 17, 2004. Despite my tendency to be obsessive-compulsive and anxious, you might expect me to have been a huge bridezilla. Surprisingly, I remained calm and relaxed throughout the entire planning process and on our special day. My mom and I had a wonderful time planning and executing the wedding, managing to do many things ourselves to save money while still achieving an elegant look and feel. Our meticulous planning allowed us to enjoy the week leading up to the wedding and the celebration itself without any last-minute rush.

The ceremony was gorgeous and full of personal touches. For instance, I walked down the aisle to *Gabriel's Oboe* from the movie The Mission, performed by my oboe teacher, Mary Beth, who is a Juilliard graduate. I have played this hauntingly beautiful piece many times, and it holds special significance for many family members. Additionally, my high school and college piano accompanist provided music during the ceremony. Both Troy and I selected pieces that were meaningful to us as a couple and held importance to me as a musician.

After the ceremony and countless photos, my parents generously allowed Troy and me to use their 1965 Ford Mustang to travel to our reception site. We stopped along the way for some intimate photos with just the two of us and our photographer. Our reception took place at a golf course supper club in a stunning, newly constructed addition. The interior featured rich, detailed woodwork, while the exterior was surrounded by lush trees and a beautifully manicured golf course. We secured an excellent deal for the entire venue, complete with a delicious and hearty meal for around 325 guests, including salad, dinner rolls, stuffed chicken, mashed potatoes with gravy, and green beans almondine.

Troy and I quickly reached an agreement on the bakery for our wedding cake, but choosing the cake's design took us quite a while. Ultimately, we decided on a simple yet elegant option, and many guests remarked that it was the best wedding cake they had ever tasted. For those curious, we managed to feed each other cake gently, avoiding any mess or cake-smashing antics. Our families found it quite bothersome to hear silverware clinking against glasses whenever guests wanted us to kiss. Nevertheless, we wanted to embrace this tradition, so we set up a miniature putting green at our reception venue. Anyone who sank a putt would prompt us to share a kiss. Additionally, we honored our venue's theme by capturing photos with our entire wedding party, as well as just the two of us, by a cluster of pine trees on the golf course. These images turned out to be some of my absolute favorites from the day.

Due to my back pain and the timing later in the day, dancing at weddings is usually a challenge for me, but I genuinely enjoyed our wedding dance. I cherished my first dance with Troy as a married couple. I also cherished the special father/daughter and mother/son dances, along with dances with family members and friends. I also loved the other memorable moments, such as Troy's dance to retrieve the garter, our grand march, and when he and his groomsmen serenaded me with *You've Lost That Lovin' Feeling*, just like in the movie *Top Gun*. We made sure to visit each table to greet our guests and express our gratitude for their presence, as we were truly touched that so many of our invited friends and family could attend. The following day, opening all the gifts from those who spent their hard-earned money on us was a bit overwhelming, but incredibly heartwarming.

Troy is truly the center of my world and the love of my life. Ever since I was a little girl, I have prayed to find him after witnessing the bond between my parents. I cherished the affection they shared, their hugs, kisses, and deep friendship, and I learned the significance of companionship in a marriage. From a young age, I recognized that this was the kind of relationship I desired with my husband. Throughout my dating journey, I never came close to finding someone who could fulfill that dream until I met Troy, who made it a reality.

I consider myself incredibly fortunate to have Troy as my husband, as he has offered me immense emotional support throughout our time together. Getting to know him over the years has been a delightful journey, as I continually discover new qualities to love about him. He always makes me feel cherished, which I deeply value since I need that validation regularly. Moreover, as our relationship progressed, it felt as if we had known each other forever. It is difficult to imagine my life before Troy; in many ways, it feels like it truly began when we became a couple. We understand each other so well, and there is a comforting ease that comes with that knowledge. I adore how sometimes words are unnecessary; a simple glance can convey our thoughts. There are even moments when Troy will say exactly what I was about to express, and the same happens in reverse.

Troy is not just an amazing husband; he is also an incredible son, uncle, nephew, cousin, friend, and all-around wonderful person. Everyone who meets him instantly takes a liking to Troy, and I feel incredibly fortunate to have married him and to enjoy all of his wonderful qualities. Troy has a fantastic sense of humor that brings me so much joy. His ability to make me laugh reminds me that not only is laughter the best medicine, but it also helps me maintain a positive, hopeful attitude. He offers me immense comfort, both verbally and physically, and is incredibly gentle and kind. In the face of life's challenges, he remains my rock and my source of strength, providing calm amidst the storms. He is undoubtedly my protector, always encouraging and supporting me when I need it most. The values of honesty and trust are paramount in our relationship, and I am grateful for how strong these qualities are between us.

Moreover, Troy is the most patient and easygoing person I have ever encountered. You may have guessed that I can be a bit more high-strung, but I believe some of his "go with the flow" attitude has rubbed off on me, making me better than I used to be. For instance, when I begin to feel overwhelmed, Troy is right there to help calm me down and offer a fresh perspective. His uncanny ability to look at me in those moments helps me regain my composure, and he gently points out alternative views on the situation.

As my back pain has intensified over the years, I find myself on the couch more frequently, feeling like a terrible, worthless wife and person. Since our marriage, my medical conditions have also multiplied in both number and severity, making me quite different from the person Troy married on that beautiful day in April 2004. I worry about how this will impact my life moving forward, but my greater concern lies with how it affects Troy. It is crucial to me that he understands just how deeply I love him and how much I appreciate everything he does for our family.

Even in times of pain and misery, I strive to accomplish as much as I can. However, I often find myself worrying about how this impacts Troy, as my thoughts sometimes drift into dark places. One of those troubling thoughts is the fear that Troy might leave me for someone who can offer him what I cannot, such as children and an active lifestyle. You may recall that when we learned I could not have biological children, I suggested that Troy consider divorcing me. He is still young enough to find another partner who could provide him with the family he deserves. I was sincere in my offer, but the mere thought of losing Troy is devastating. Ultimately, I was trying to prioritize his happiness. Our friends and family reassured me that I was being irrational to think Troy would not want to stay with me, and I believe I understood that, too.

Troy and I are deeply in love, and he supports me wholeheartedly, both in my health and in my endeavors with my book and nonprofit work. Still, I felt compelled to make the offer to reassure myself that Troy would remain committed to our marriage, no matter what.

When we exchanged vows on April 17, 2004, we pledged to support each other "in good times and in bad, in sickness and in health." These vows hold significant meaning for us, and I'm incredibly fortunate that Troy loves me more than he longs for the idea of finding someone else and having children. A crucial element of marriage is communication, which is why Troy and I openly discussed our inability to have children and how it has affected our plans. Effective communication is essential to a successful relationship. With the various challenges we face, particularly medical ones, we recognize that maintaining solid and regular communication is vital.

While I may be limited physically and unable to give Troy everything he deserves, like children, our deep love for each other is what truly matters. Moreover, I am immensely grateful for everything Troy does for me and our family, and I feel blessed to have his love. Most importantly, I want to express my deep regret that I cannot give Troy children. However, I am immensely grateful for everything he does to care for me and our cat each day. I strive to contribute as much as I can by paying the bills and balancing the checkbook, making appointments, helping keep the house clean, and any other tasks that I can tackle. Yet, I have my limitations and cannot do it all, so I want Troy to know just how thankful I am for his unwavering support. I truly feel like the luckiest girl in the world to have him in my life. He cares for me with such a positive attitude, capturing my heart and soul entirely. I cherish our time together and am incredibly grateful that we are not just a loving couple, but also wonderful friends.

Although we are unable to have our own biological children, we have decided to be pet parents, and we are fortunate to currently have a delightful cat. In the past, we have also shared our lives with some amazing felines, too. Adapting our life plan to exclude having biological children has been challenging, but what matters most is that Troy and I have each other. Our marriage is strong, filled with love and companionship.

Marriage is a journey with its highs and lows, filled with joyous moments as well as challenges. It's how we respond to these situations that teaches us valuable lessons and shapes the course of our relationship. I would say that many of our struggles have centered around medical conditions and their lasting effects. Very few people understand the full extent of these issues and their significant impact on various aspects of life. The dreams we had when we married in 2004 have had to change dramatically, and the financial, emotional, physical, and social challenges could easily strain a marriage. This is not a common experience for most couples, but Troy has navigated it all with grace. He has cared for me selflessly, without complaint, and has adjusted to every obstacle in the most supportive and unselfish way.

My Parents:

I am extremely close to my parents. Everything I experienced as a young child diagnosed with cancer, followed by my journey as a childhood cancer survivor, truly united us. I feel incredibly fortunate to have survived, surrounded by their unwavering love and support. Our family has always been tightly knit, and our closeness has continued to grow and evolve. Even now, I speak with both of my parents every day. They have been remarkable parents to my brother and me, serving as wonderful friends and essential pillars of support throughout my childhood and into adulthood.

Our family's closeness has not gone unnoticed, which is a wonderful compliment. For instance, during church services, we would often huddle together, sometimes holding hands in the pews. One Sunday, a fellow congregant approached us and expressed how much they admired the warmth radiating from our family. What a heartfelt and meaningful compliment! Honestly, I believe that our bond might not be as strong as it is today had I not faced cancer. I like to think of this as one of the silver linings of my cancer journey, if one can truly find a silver lining in such an experience.

My parents are the most selfless people that I have ever met. They would do anything for anyone, and I have witnessed their kindness countless times. For instance, if a neighbor requires their lawn to be mowed, they will step in without hesitation, regardless of the personal cost. Despite having their own aches, pains, and medical issues, my parents willingly set aside their discomfort to assist others, including my husband and me. They often lend a hand with our lawn care, particularly during the fall when our yard is overwhelmed with leaves. Unfortunately, my husband is usually tasked with managing the lawn, especially when it comes to raking and clearing the abundant fall foliage. Without fail, my parents are there to help tackle the leaf collection and prepare our yard and plants for winter.

Additionally, they offer support with household chores and various projects that arise. They have also provided us financial assistance on numerous occasions, often without us even needing to ask. While I feel guilty about relying on their help, I am profoundly grateful for all the support they have given my husband and me throughout our marriage.

One of the greatest gifts my brother and I received from our parents was the example of a loving marriage and a genuine friendship that we aspired to emulate. Growing up, I always envisioned a relationship like theirs, filled with the love they shared for each other and our family. They faced numerous trials and challenges that tested their marriage, challenges that could have easily shattered their bond. You may recall the storybook couple introduced at the beginning of this book, who seemed so deeply in love at the start of their journey. Often, marriages crumble under the strain of circumstances like childhood cancer, yet my parents' love only deepened over the years, and their relationship became even stronger. This transformation did not come without effort; they will readily attest to the hard work it required. Remarkably, the love depicted in the opening of this book only multiplied, evolving my parents' relationship into something even more exquisite. They are truly best friends and partners in love, and I take immense pride in the bond they have nurtured. I am also thankful for the wonderful example of love and friendship they provided, which, as you have read, has greatly influenced my own relationship with my husband. Additionally, the loving connections we share as a family are incredibly special, and I believe they may not have been as strong if I had not faced cancer.

Gabriel ("Gabe"), My Brother:

Although my brother, Gabriel, is five years younger than I, and I spent many years babysitting and caring for him, he has now taken on the role of a protective older brother, doing the kindest things to look after me. Facing a cancer diagnosis and undergoing treatment was incredibly tough, but siblings often bear the weight of childhood cancer and are regarded as the silent victims of pediatric cancer. My dad even wrote his thesis for his master's degree in psychology on this very subject, referring to them as the "forgotten ones." Erma Bombeck touches on this issue in her book, I Want to Grow Hair, I Want to Grow Up, I Want to Go to Boise. This book is quite dated, and I turned to it during my own childhood, yet it still remains relevant today. One significant concern for siblings when their brother or sister is diagnosed with cancer is the feeling of guilt, as they may mistakenly believe that they are somehow responsible for the illness. They often reflect on past misbehavior and think that their sibling's cancer is a form of punishment. Additionally, they worry about the possibility of developing cancer themselves. Siblings frequently endure these and other challenges while their brother or sister undergoes treatment. Additionally, these siblings may experience challenges such as developing physical symptoms to seek attention, declining grades in school, suppressed emotions, feeling fear, resentment, confusion, shame, jealousy, embarrassment, and apprehension.

Furthermore, siblings of childhood cancer patients often find themselves shuffled between various homes, longing to be in their own space with their family. While it is usually essential for parents to stay with the sick child, healthy siblings may need to reside with friends or relatives. Moreover, they frequently lack updates about their sibling's condition, which can lead to unnecessary worry and create a distorted perception that may be worse than the reality.

At its core, childhood cancer affects every aspect of a family's life and each family member. In the journal article, *Siblings' Experiences with Childhood Cancer: A Different Way of Being in the Family*, Roberta Lynn Woodgate elaborates that for siblings, "cancer was experienced as a different way of being within their family and involved siblings undergoing a loss of a family way of life and a loss of self within the family." Three key themes emerged regarding this altered family dynamic: committing to keeping the family together, being present, and enduring sadness. This highlights the urgent need for additional support for healthy siblings in families affected by childhood cancer. It truly saddens me to think of any child experiencing these feelings, especially at such a young age during a time of family turmoil.

You might be curious why I am addressing this topic when my brother was born five years after me and four years after my diagnosis. The reason is that I faced late effects, surgeries, and numerous doctor appointments due to my cancer, and my brother had to navigate this reality from birth. This situation resonates not only with siblings of childhood cancer patients but also with those siblings having any type of illness, including late effects and medical conditions related to childhood cancer. My brother endured all these emotions as I was the ill child, while he was the healthy one experiencing the challenges described above. He has expressed that he felt compelled to behave perfectly to avoid adding unnecessary worry for our parents, who already had plenty on their plates with my health issues. This thought deeply saddens me, knowing my brother was born into a life filled with my medical challenges; I can only imagine how young he was when he first began to feel this way. My parents were acutely aware of this potential dynamic, which is why they chose to wait so long between my birth and his. They wanted me to be finished with my cancer treatments before having him. Little did they know I would face a multitude of late effects and medical issues long after my treatments concluded.

Despite having these feelings, my brother and I were very close growing up. I babysat him all the time, so playing together just became a natural thing for the two of us to do. Given the age gap between us, I became like a second mother to Gabe. Yet, I learned that Gabe was still protective of me when we were younger. I did not know the extent of this until I was older, but I guess kids on the school bus used to make fun of me for wearing my pants high on my waist. Part of this was because I had a high waist, but the other part of it was because of the back brace. Gabe used to stand up for me when kids would tease me behind my back about this, so that I would not hear their comments and feel bad. As we grew older, our relationship shifted, and I had to learn how to become more of a friend to Gabe, as opposed to a babysitter/second mother. This took some adjustment for both of us, but we eventually became good friends, and I can wholeheartedly say that my brother is one of my best friends.

My brother has also promised my parents that he would take care of me if they are gone and my husband could no longer do so. This brings tears to my eyes because my brother grew up feeling like the "forgotten one" at certain times in his life. He is also my younger brother, so I should be taking care of him and not the other way around. Yet, he has fully promised to take care of me, cementing his role as a protective brother. I think back to that day in the car after my appointment when I was told that I would have back pain for the rest of my life. He was so young at that time, yet he knew how to take care of me in that moment. I am so blessed that he has agreed to continue to take care of me, and that he just inherently does so. It seems to come naturally to him, and for that I am also very grateful.

Beyond our friendship and sibling bond, I take immense pride in my brother for several reasons. He holds a degree in business management and has successfully ascended to the position of store manager at a high-volume Ulta location. In this role, he oversees the entire store, ensuring that every employee is valued and treated with respect and kindness. Ulta is committed to diversity in its workforce. For instance, they hire men and drag queens who excel in makeup application. My brother even had the honor of speaking at Ulta's national conference one year, showcasing the diverse and appreciated team at his store.

He diligently reviews all financial documents related to both his store and Ulta overall, often worrying about how his store is performing. At times, this dedication leads him to bring work home, but this demonstrates his deep commitment to his job, his employees, and the company as a whole.

Our phone conversations are always filled with joy, as we dive into discussions about makeup, hair, and skincare, indulging our passions. He can effortlessly answer any question I have regarding the best products to use or whether a particular item is worth the investment. The excitement of these conversations is mutual. I genuinely value his insights and hang on to every word of his advice. I believe he enjoys these chats as well, often asking about my thoughts on new products he recommends.

In addition to his professional achievements, I am incredibly proud of my brother on a personal level. When he was in his early twenties, he courageously came to terms with his identity as a gay man. I admired his bravery in sharing this with us, and it did not alter the love and support our family had for him. My hopes remained the same. I wished for him to find a partner akin to Troy or my dad. He ultimately found that in a wonderful man named Jason, and they quickly fell in love and became a couple. They eventually moved in together and adopted two cats. I think my parents are destined to be cat grandparents!

In 2022, Gabe and Jason tied the knot, and we had an absolute blast celebrating their wedding. Our family has embraced Jason wholeheartedly, and we take pride in him as an individual, as well as in their partnership. Beyond witnessing the beautiful love they share, both Gabe and Jason are incredibly philanthropic, generous, kind, and supportive. They bring so much laughter and joy into our lives.

My Cats:

Animals, especially my cherished pets, play a vital role in my "Inner Circle." Their comfort, companionship, and unconditional love have been invaluable to me, particularly during the long hours I spend alone at home while my husband is at work. Yet, I am never truly alone, as there is always a cat by my side. Typically, I am lying on the couch and working on my laptop, with my cat, Isaac, curled up next to me. In the evenings, our positions shift, and Isaac often lies on top of me, encouraging me to heed my doctor's advice and take a break to rest completely.

Boots, Morris, and Dolce

The bond between humans and animals is profound, and we often regard our pets as family members. This bond began with our first indoor cats, Boots and Morris, whom my brother and I adopted in elementary school, and it has only strengthened with each new cat. After losing Boots to stomach cancer, I rescued a tiny kitten from the animal shelter and named her Dolce, a musical term meaning "sweetly."

I had Dolce through many key moments in my life, starting the summer before 8th grade, a tough year marked by exclusion and depression. She stayed by my side through high school, college, law school, business school, and the early years of my marriage to Troy. Her presence during these pivotal times made her an incredibly special companion. As my first adult pet, our bond was strengthened by my sole responsibility for her care. Dolce was attentive, always coming when I called, and brought comfort during hard times. She slept by my side each night, offering steady companionship. Though she was a one-person cat who treasured our time together, she eventually became a two-person cat, growing to love Troy, too, almost as if giving him her stamp of approval.

Isaac and Holly

Losing Dolce to kidney disease and heart problems was incredibly painful, but I knew I needed another feline companion. I soon fell for Isaac, a seal-point Siamese with icy blue, crossed eyes, at the animal shelter where I volunteered. Once a stray, he arrived sick and scarred, with dull, sticky fur and healing burns on his legs and feet, likely from a car engine. His tail hung broken, his toe was twisted, and one nail curved unnaturally upward. Despite it all, he had a sweet soul and a strong spirit.

When I found myself calling Isaac "my cat," I adopted him without hesitation. We chose August 12, his adoption day, as his birthday. Isaac's intelligent, playful Siamese nature quickly became apparent, knocking items off tables, biting paperwork, and chasing balls. Though clumsy from his cross-eyed vision, he loved attention, responded to his name, and even walked well on a leash until age slowed him down. Now 19, he's still a loyal, affectionate companion who curls up beside me and lifts my spirits every day.

Knowing Siamese cats bond deeply, we adopted a second cat, Holly. I met her in 2010, soon after losing Dolce. She reminded me of Dolce, which made me hesitate at first. Labeled "unadoptable" for her extreme shyness, Holly needed someone patient and kind. I had worked with many shy cats, and our connection was immediate. She purred and let me scratch her belly the first time I met her, the ultimate sign of trust!

We brought her home on February 9, 2011, but chose February 6, when the Packers won the Super Bowl, as her birthday. Holly was terrified at first and would sometimes lose control of her bladder from fear. We brought home a shelter cage to help her transition and gradually built her confidence. Over time, she began eating, playing, and sleeping outside the cage. Isaac helped her learn how to play and feel safe again, while Holly taught him boundaries and grooming. They formed a beautiful bond.

Though small, we suspected Holly had Maine Coon heritage: silky long fur, snowshoe paws, and the classic "M" on her forehead. She was sweet and intelligent, loved quietly observing, and followed us around the house. She disliked change but adored our friend Gavin, my husband Troy, and me. Holly's final years were hard and consisted of fluid in her lungs, steroids, steroids, and diabetes, but we cherished every moment. When the time came, we held her, whispering love as she passed peacefully in our arms.

Holly and Isaac became our family. We couldn't have children, so they filled that space with unconditional love. As someone who is often homebound with medical challenges, their companionship meant everything. They became my comfort, my night nurses, my joy. Isaac turned 19 in 2025 and remains by my side, sensing when I'm upset and offering quiet comfort.

Through them, I've learned patience, strength, and the power of love without conditions. They never asked me to change and loved me just as I am. Even in grief, I am filled with gratitude for the joy they brought and the resilience they showed. Their love has made me a better, stronger person, and I will carry their lessons in my heart forever.

Gavin:

I feel incredibly lucky and recognize my good fortune for the people and experiences in my life and what I have overcome. I am blessed to have met and married my loving husband, Troy, and I have a wonderfully close-knit family through marriage. Now, in my mid-40s, I have cultivated several quality friendships that enrich my "Inner Circle."

Gavin is a true friend I can rely on completely and share my thoughts with, allowing us to discuss nearly anything. I met Gavin while volunteering at the animal shelter where I adopted Holly and Isaac. My role at the shelter involved volunteering during and after office hours, as well as assisting with cat adoptions. I was also honored to be elected to the Board of Directors, where I contributed by writing the shelter's newsletter, a weekly "Pet of the Week" feature, and other necessary content.

I initially connected with Gavin and his wife through email. They dedicated their time to cleaning the shelter's isolation room several times a week and took stunning, professional-quality photos of the cats to enhance their chances of adoption. A captivating image can significantly increase a cat's likelihood of being adopted, making their efforts invaluable. Furthermore, Gavin took on the responsibility of managing the shelter's website, which required me to frequently communicate with him and share the articles I had written for posting.

As we worked together at the animal shelter, Gavin and I formed a deep friendship, bonding especially over our shared love for helping shy cats. Over the years, we met regularly and grew incredibly in tune with each other. Gavin can often read my thoughts or sense my pain just by looking at me. He's a deeply intuitive and caring person and has gone above and beyond to help me, even researching treatments for my complex medical issues.

Importantly, Gavin is one of only three people my cat fully trusts. He takes wonderful care of Isaac when Troy and I are away, which gives me peace of mind. He sends me updates and pictures without hesitation, knowing how much it means to me. It might seem small to others, but those updates help me feel close to Isaac and remind me how lucky I am to have a friend like Gavin.

One quality I truly value is how deeply Gavin cares about all my medical issues. He consistently keeps track of my doctor appointments and eagerly asks about how they go. When I undergo surgery or any significant procedure, he is always one of the first people I reach out to afterward, to let him know that I'm doing well. Moreover, Gavin frequently researches online to gain a better understanding of my medical conditions. He actively seeks out new treatments or ideas that could benefit me, while also identifying things to avoid that might harm me.

Gavin and I have been friends since 2010, and I feel grateful and fortunate to have him in my life. He has taught me the true meaning of friendship and has proven that genuine friends do exist.

Diana:

My friendship with Diana is relatively new compared to some of my other friends and members of my "Inner Circle." We first met at church, where we both sang as sopranos in the choir. Diana moved to this area from Georgia to be closer to her son, and Good Shepherd Lutheran Church was blessed to gain her as a member. I love listening to Diana talk with her Southern accent and colloquialisms.

Diana always radiated warmth, happiness, and kindness; she would ask how I was doing and genuinely lean in to hear my response. I could sense that she truly cared, especially on days when I felt a bit more sore than usual. She would go out of her way to extend a helping hand and offer an extra smile.

Our friendship blossomed during our visits to Starbucks after church and choir rehearsals, where we engaged in wonderful, deep conversations. Those outings soon turned into even more time spent together, and before long, we became fast friends.

Diana and I have shared countless conversations throughout our friendship, which has allowed us to connect on a profound level in a relatively short time. Whether we are shopping, enjoying a meal, or simply hanging out and chatting, we always have a blast together. One of my favorite things about our friendship is how much we have fun and laugh together. Time flies by, and our enjoyment remains constant, no matter the activity. One of our favorite activities is shopping at thrift stores and finding excellent deals. I also cherish our discussions about religion and faith, and I have learned so much from Diana on these topics. Moreover, we can truly talk about anything, which is such an important quality to have in a member of my "Inner Circle."

Carolyn:

Carolyn is a fellow long-term childhood cancer survivor with over 30 years of survivorship. We first met at the Coalition Against Childhood Cancer (CAC2) Annual Summit in Columbus, Ohio, in 2019. This was the first CAC2 Annual Summit that either of us had attended, and it was particularly meaningful for Carolyn, as she grew up in Columbus.

At the Summit, we were introduced, and our connection blossomed into a wonderful friendship. Despite having different types of childhood cancer, neuroblastoma and acute lymphocytic leukemia, and being diagnosed at vastly different ages (one year old and 13 years old), we discovered that we shared many common experiences.

We both felt a deep understanding of each other as long-term survivors. We expressed how valuable it was to have someone to talk to, especially since connections and resources had been limited or nonexistent throughout much of our lives. Having grown up as survivors who often had to navigate our journeys alone, finding someone to relate to was a refreshing and incredible experience for both of us.

Not only did we develop a wonderful friendship, but we also developed a pediatric cancer survivorship program together. Better Together was started on the foundation that we are "Better Together," and we wanted to make sure that other survivors, their families, and the professionals who work with this population had access to organizations that offered current survivorship programs, support, and assistance. We both agreed that we did not want current survivors and their families to go through what we did and experience loneliness, isolation, and a lack of resources.

Sarah:

Sarah is an incredibly special friend, but unfortunately, I have never met her in person. We were introduced by a mutual acquaintance, who thought we had a lot in common and would become good friends...and she was correct! Sarah and I have had many long telephone conversations, as well as virtual meet-ups. In addition, Sarah joined the Coalition Against Childhood Cancer (CAC2), the nonprofit organization where I am the Survivorship lead, and she has helped with several of my projects and programs.

Sarah is a fellow neuroblastoma survivor, and her tumor was also located in her thoracic spinal area. In addition to neuroblastoma, she also developed leukemia from her treatments and beat it, as well as a disease in her brain called toxoplasmosis when she was going through treatments and had a weakened immune system. In addition, Sarah developed many late effects from both neuroblastoma and leukemia. We have a few late effects in common, such as: adrenal insufficiency disease; chronic, severe pain that continues to worsen each year; and gastroparesis, to name just a few. To make things interesting, we also have vastly different late effects, as well. It is incredibly easy for Sarah and me to discuss our medical issues with each other because we truly understand each other and what it is like to have a plethora of late effects from childhood cancer and its accompanying treatments.

Sarah truly embodies *hope over despair*. Sarah has had a difficult home life and has had to take care of herself for the most part since childhood. Furthermore, despite having a ton of medical conditions and experiencing cancer twice in her life, Sarah maintains the best, positive, hopeful attitude. She also influences those around her to have the same outlook on life, and it is difficult to be sad or negative when you are around Sarah. I am so incredibly proud of Sarah and all that she has overcome, while still maintaining a wonderful attitude and sense of humor.

All of these wonderful people, and my cat, Isaac, make up my current "Inner Circle", and I can talk to them about anything. I often discuss difficult times with my medical issues because they are the only ones who know the true extent of this part of my life. I also have a difficult time sharing these feelings with others for a variety of reasons, such as fear of sounding like I am complaining, or someone not understanding the childhood cancer experience, and thinking that I was incredibly strange, having so many medical conditions. Yet, no matter what I throw at them, my "Inner Circle" continues to love and support me, and they are a definite "must" for me to continue to pursue hope, optimism, and positivity in my life.

Music as an Outlet

Having a hobby or a passion that you genuinely enjoy is vital for fostering hope, optimism, and positivity. Personally, I have never been graceful or athletic. While I did join the women's golf team as a freshman and sophomore in high school, my skills were lacking, and I had to stop playing after injuring my back during a meet. It's believed that this injury occurred because I was permitted to remove my back brace while golfing. My back muscles had weakened while in the brace, and the repetitive, forceful action of a golf swing ultimately proved too much for them, resulting in tears.

Following my parents' advice, I also attempted to join the long-distance running team in junior high P.E., but that was another unfortunate experience. I was lapped multiple times and consistently finished in last place. My parents now openly acknowledge that they were mistaken in encouraging me to participate in extracurricular sports, particularly distance running. Despite these challenges, I still needed to put forth significant effort in Physical Education class, as it was part of my overall grade, and I did not want it to jeopardize my chances of becoming valedictorian.

Yet, my parents wanted to put me in some sort of extracurricular activity, so they enrolled me in piano lessons when I was in 2nd grade, which was the earliest that my first piano teacher would allow students to enroll. That turned out to be an excellent idea because I loved music, and I made sure that I practiced every single day. I progressed and advanced quite quickly, and I was really happy learning how to play the piano.

This first piano teacher taught me for a few years, but she eventually cut back on teaching, so I started taking piano lessons from a different piano teacher who was quite accomplished and popular within the area. I took lessons with her throughout high school, until I stopped taking piano lessons altogether when I left to go to college.

When I got to high school, I began accompanying the choir, show choir, and individuals competing with an instrument or singing vocals in Solo and Ensemble, a yearly "competition" that would give instrumental and vocal awards to individuals and groups in various levels of musical difficulty. I quickly progressed to the most advanced level of music, received first place in many of them, and also went to State to play or sing my solos each year. Also, I had always been a singer, but I started to study it and sing in Solo and Ensemble around the time that I was in junior high. I was a soprano and could hit fairly high notes. (Even today, I can still hit almost all of the high notes in our church choir pieces.)

In 5th grade, my classmates and I had the opportunity to choose instruments that we could learn to play for 5th grade band. I actually wanted to play a string instrument, but since my schools did not offer orchestra, I opted for the flute instead. I began private lessons in 6th grade with our outstanding junior high band director and quickly improved, eventually playing alongside talented 8th graders. By 8th grade, I was briefly first chair, but I struggled with breathing due to asthma and restrictive lung disease, which limited my right lung's capacity. Despite practicing both flute and piano daily, my breathing challenges made progress with the flute difficult and frustrating.

Midway through 8th grade, the high school band teacher approached me about switching from flute to oboe. She explained that there would be many flutists in high school and that I was too strong a musician to get lost in the section. I was unfamiliar with the oboe but pretended I knew what it was, then researched it and decided to give it a try. At first, I was unable to make a sound, mainly because she forgot to include a reed with the instrument! Even with the reed, however, it was difficult, but I was determined. I accepted her offer, and we agreed that I would play the piccolo for marching and pep band, which was an honor because only the best flutists were allowed to play the piccolo. In addition, I began private oboe lessons, which my parents supported. That marked the beginning of my ongoing journey with the oboe.

Since my parents did not know any oboists, they reached out to musicians in our network and eventually connected with Mary Beth, the principal oboist of the La Crosse Symphony Orchestra and a graduate of the prestigious, world-class Juilliard School, specializing in dance, drama, and music. After speaking with her about my dedication to music and my background in flute, which shares similar fingerings with oboe, she agreed to take me on as a student. At my first lesson, I still couldn't produce a sound. Mary Beth explained how sensitive oboe reeds are and the importance of soaking them and choosing the right brand. After learning how to properly form my embouchure, I was finally able to get a sound out and begin learning the notes.

From 8th grade through my senior year, I traveled 27 miles one way for weekly oboe lessons with Mary Beth. I began with lesson books and gradually advanced to more challenging material, practicing at least 45 minutes daily. By the end of 8th grade, I felt confident on the oboe and ready for high school. Music became my refuge, a place where I felt I belonged and could truly excel, especially after struggling in sports. Before I could drive, my parents took me to lessons, and once I had my permit, I practiced driving that familiar route. The trips became valuable bonding time with my family, full of shared stories and conversations. Sometimes, a parent would drive while I finished homework; other times, they'd run errands and return just in time. Those drives shaped both my musical journey and my driving skills.

I attended college fairly locally in La Crosse, Wisconsin. Mary Beth was employed as a music professor there, so that meant that I could continue to take lessons from her throughout my time in college. Lessons were just one credit, so I always had room in my schedule for them. I studied with Mary Beth once a week from 8th grade all the way through my 3½ years of undergraduate studies.

One challenge I have faced in playing oboe and singing is chronic dry mouth. Since oboists constantly soak their reeds to keep them playable, dryness can be a real obstacle, just as it is for singers. I manage it by staying hydrated, using dry mouth sprays, getting fluoride treatments, chewing gum in between playing the oboe, and frequently rewetting my reed. Despite the inconvenience, my love for music far outweighs the challenge. Interestingly, unlike the flute, the oboe requires less air but more control, which suited my lung condition better. As previously discussed, my pulmonologist even noted improved breathing tests over time, likely because oboe playing strengthened my respiratory muscles.

Music has always been my primary form of self-expression, and sometimes I do not know how to express myself any other way. Whether I'm playing classical pieces, marching band music, or listening to my favorite songs, music is constantly in my head and heart. During brief times when I have stepped away from the oboe, I felt incomplete, as if something essential was missing. Music has given me both a sense of belonging and an individual pursuit where I can grow and succeed. It became my own version of a "team sport," and most of my closest friendships have been rooted in our shared love of music.

Throughout high school and college, I performed in many ensembles, including the college orchestra, which aided me in meeting my husband. Today, I continue playing the oboe in community groups and at church, and I sing soprano in the church choir. The oboe remains my primary instrument and first love, offering me a way to express emotions and connect with others. I strive for my audience to truly feel the music I play. Even though I experience pain while playing, I choose to keep doing what I love because music keeps me going. It's how I live with a song in both my head and my heart.

Gratitude, Kindness, and Giving Back

My medical issues and other experiences have helped mold me into the person that I am today. Although my medical problems take up a significant portion of my life, they do not represent my entire life. I have purposefully cultivated a life with incredibly meaningful work that I am fully passionate about, but that still allows me to lie down on the couch with my laptop to work, with my Siamese cat, Isaac, by my side. I can also create my own schedule to give me the rest that I need, to attend doctor appointments regularly, and to space out my activities so that I can build recovery time into my schedule. My nonprofit work has also given me incredible gratitude and a desire to help more childhood cancer patients, survivors, and their families. I have learned so much from this work, which has fully enriched my life.

Furthermore, for me, practicing gratitude and perpetuating kindness is so important, and I do this through my work with several different nonprofits that include neuroblastoma and childhood cancer organizations, as well as general cancer-related nonprofits. I had some amazing experiences doing this work, and I finally feel like I am doing what I am supposed to be doing with my life. I want to use my experiences with having cancer to help families, patients, and survivors, and to fight childhood cancer in a variety of ways. Childhood cancer research gets very little funding, and that tiny bit of funding needs to be divided among the 16 different types of childhood cancer and hundreds of subtypes.

Awareness of the different types of childhood cancer and their prevalence is also important. In several of my organizations, I help raise funds for both childhood cancer research and awareness. Through my work, I also talk with people currently facing childhood cancer, as well as survivors, and I do research for various organizations. I lead the childhood cancer survivorship portion of an international nonprofit, and this group and I have developed two exciting survivorship programs. I am also working on various projects with other organizations. I got to speak at a national neuroblastoma conference, and I have written various articles and other pieces. I have had many other unique, rewarding experiences that I will touch upon in this section, but honestly, just being a part of all of these organizations and getting to do the important work surrounding childhood cancer is enough of a reward for me.

My nonprofit work truly fulfills me and gives me a sense of purpose. One of my key desires and goals in life has been to fight neuroblastoma and all childhood cancers, and to help patients, survivors, and families feel less alone and isolated, because that has been a battle for my parents and me, especially when I was younger. For current and future patients and survivors, I would love to make things at least a little easier than what my family and I endured. Additionally, helping others is so important, and my work with these nonprofits provides me with gratitude and a sense of purpose. It helps get me outside of my own life and difficulties, as well as my pain and many medical issues, and it allows me to use my experiences to help people. I have had some amazing experiences fighting cancer with these organizations, and I have a spot in my heart for each one.

I am active in 5-10 different nonprofits at a time, and they are related to neuroblastoma, childhood cancer, and cancer in general. Through this work, I try to communicate with as many families, patients, and survivors as I can, offering comfort and words of support, discussing my personal experiences, conducting research, and in any other ways that I can help. I like to stress that I am not a medical professional. Rather, I have just been in clinics and hospitals throughout my entire life, and I have a lot of medical conditions, have been involved with many different specialties, have had a lot of procedures, and I have had 52 surgeries. Additionally, I have done some motivational/inspirational speaking, and I truly hope that this book will help the childhood cancer community. I created a website (www.HopeOverDespair.com) with the hope of selling my book and creating more speaking opportunities in the future. Overall, I have a sense of purpose and am very passionate and fulfilled by this work. It truly fills my heart and soul to fight for past, present, and future children who are fighting neuroblastoma and other childhood cancers.

Neuroblastoma Children's Cancer Society:

I began my nonprofit work by contacting a small neuroblastoma nonprofit, the Neuroblastoma Children's Cancer Society (NCCS), and asking them if I could help in any way. They seemed very grateful for the help, and this started the beginning of a beautiful relationship. The Sexton family is incredibly giving, generous, and caring, and they have truly made me feel like a member of the family.

At the age of 2½, Michael Sexton courageously battled neuroblastoma, but his fight tragically ended nine months later, one month after his third birthday. After Michael died, his parents, Jim and Dori Sexton, were shocked to learn that no major organizations were funding significant research to promote a frontline treatment or a cure for neuroblastoma. In honor of Michael and other children who died of neuroblastoma, the NCCS was formed in 1994. The mission is to cure neuroblastoma and its related childhood cancers, as well as to improve the quality of life for patients, survivors, and their families. This is accomplished by raising funds to support researchers investigating the causes, treatments, and cures for neuroblastoma and related cancers. Other vital components of our mission are generating public awareness and providing support, resources, and assistance to the neuroblastoma community. Finally, we advocate for government research funding and associated public policies for all types of childhood cancers.

The NCCS donates almost all of its revenue to research because childhood cancers are vastly and consistently underfunded, so it falls to private organizations to fill in the funding gaps and pay for this desperately needed research. Most of us in this community are probably familiar with the "More than 4" slogan, which was used to refer to the approximately 4% of the cancer research budget that the federal government donated to all types of childhood cancer research. That number has been increasing, however, and it may be closer to 8% depending on the numbers being used in the calculations. Yet, it still does not seem like enough, especially when you consider that certain types of childhood cancer have a virtually 0% survival rate, and chemotherapy medications have remained the same for decades. For example, three of the four chemotherapy medications that I had are still being used to treat neuroblastoma today, more than 45 years after I received them. It is my understanding that the 4th chemotherapy medication has been deemed too dangerous for neuroblastoma treatments on young children. Additionally, remember that the total amount given by the federal government to childhood cancer research needs to be divided among all of the 16 types of childhood cancer and hundreds of subtypes.

Not only do we need to bring up the survival rate for neuroblastoma, but we need better, less toxic treatments so that we can decrease the number and severity of late effects for survivors. Finally, neuroblastoma also has a high rate of relapse, and there are no standard treatments for relapsed neuroblastoma. Instead, each child receives individualized treatments and is often entered into clinical trials. Since NCCS originated in 1994, we have formed partnerships and donated more than $2 million to researchers at various hospitals, including the Children's Hospital of Los Angeles and the Children's Hospital of Philadelphia. The majority of our research funding, however, has been donated to the University of Chicago for various neuroblastoma research grants and to help support the Pediatric Cancer Data Commons (PCDC), which holds pediatric, AYA, and adult clinical data for various types of cancers, but the focus has been on pediatric cancers and originated with clinical data for neuroblastoma.

Various types of support and services are also crucial for childhood cancer patients, families, and survivors, and NCCS is there for them in several different ways. For example, we offer a variety of resources and educational tools because families facing childhood cancer are often overwhelmed by the sheer amount of information they must absorb in a short amount of time. Knowledge and education are very important when understanding what is happening with the diagnosis, treatment, and survival of neuroblastoma, so we want to make things a little easier by providing information all in one place. That way, they do not have to search for information on their own, and it is all housed in one area for families to refer to when needed. We also believe it is important to provide various types of support networks and assistance to neuroblastoma patients, families, and survivors, and we provide this through: our private Facebook group; our Facebook, Twitter, and Instagram accounts; our website; and our membership in the Coalition Against Childhood Cancer. As more patients and families face neuroblastoma or a related childhood cancer diagnosis, and as others move toward survivorship, we want those in our community to be aware of NCCS so that we can help even more people.

<u>American Cancer Society Cancer Action Network</u>:

I joined the American Cancer Society Cancer Action Network (ACS CAN) after several years of independently advocating for childhood cancer awareness and funding. At the time, Congress was considering the STAR Act (Survivorship, Treatment, Access, and Research), a major childhood cancer bill. I had contacted the federal Senators and Representatives from Wisconsin on my own, but could not secure a meeting. Then I came across ACS CAN on Facebook and learned they were a well-respected organization with strong connections to lawmakers. After researching them further, I realized my advocacy efforts would have a greater impact through ACS CAN.

ACS CAN is the nonprofit, nonpartisan advocacy affiliate of the American Cancer Society and the nation's leading cancer advocacy group. It works with elected officials at both the state and federal levels to prioritize the needs of cancer patients and survivors through policy change. Among its many achievements, ACS CAN helped pass the STAR Act on June 5, 2018, and continues to secure its annual funding. The STAR Act remains the most comprehensive childhood cancer legislation to date.

ACS CAN equips new volunteers with the tools and training to become effective advocates. Volunteers can participate at whatever level they choose, from promoting campaigns on social media and collecting petitions, to contacting lawmakers, attending events, writing letters to the editor, or fundraising. With ACS CAN's support, every volunteer can find their voice and make a difference.

If volunteers choose to advocate directly with legislators and their staff, ACS CAN provides full training to prepare them. Volunteers do not need to be policy experts, just experts on their own stories. These personal stories are powerful and memorable, often making the biggest impact during meetings with lawmakers.

One of the most rewarding parts of being involved with ACS CAN is meeting people with powerful stories and diverse backgrounds. Some joined because of a loved one with cancer, others as caregivers, and many as survivors themselves. Despite our varied reasons for joining, we all share a passion for fighting cancer and making a difference.

I've been an ACS CAN advocate since 2017 and have had the privilege of many unique and meaningful experiences. I've built relationships with both state and federal legislators and participated in lobby and action days, including ACS CAN's Summit and Leadership Lobby Day, the Alliance for Childhood Cancer Action Days, One Voice Against Cancer (OVAC), and more. I've also written several letters to the editor from 2018 to 2023 and was honored to contribute a guest post to the ACS CAN national website about my childhood cancer advocacy.

In 2019, I delivered a legislative briefing at the U.S. Capitol on the six protected classes of medications. Since then, I have had multiple speaking engagements for ACS CAN on various healthcare initiatives. I have spoken with the press, both in print and on television, about ACS CAN and our legislative priorities, including in The New York Times on Medicare Part D coverage. I also appeared in a national commercial in 2019 about the six protected medications, which aired on social media and D.C. television markets. One especially fun highlight was having a full film crew at my home, complete with hair and makeup.

Through these experiences, I've learned how powerful sharing my story can be. As an ACS CAN volunteer, I truly feel heard. It's an honor to speak with legislators and advocate on behalf of current and future cancer patients and survivors. I carry with me the voices of childhood cancer patients, survivors, and angels, past, present, and future. I hope that my work helps increase awareness and drive meaningful legislative change.

Wisconsin Cancer Collaborative:

In 2023, I expanded my state-level advocacy by joining the Wisconsin Cancer Collaborative. While in Washington, D.C., I met Autumn Gentry, a new CAC2 member and fellow Wisconsinite. Autumn, a bereaved parent who lost her daughter Isla to acute myeloid leukemia (AML), now works in childhood cancer advocacy through the MACC Fund (Midwest Athletes Against Childhood Cancer). I was inspired by her strength and dedication. Together, we helped develop and create a pediatric cancer action plan for Wisconsin and advocate to ensure childhood cancer is included in the state's revised cancer plan for 2030–2040.

We attended the 2023 Wisconsin Cancer Summit and met two wonderful people from the Wisconsin Cancer Collaborative: Beth Brunner, the Program Director, and Alexandria Cull Weatherer, an Outreach Specialist. Together, we created the Wisconsin Pediatric Cancer Action Plan, 2024-2028. The purpose of this plan is to fill "the gaps found within the awareness, education, and care given to those with cancer as children," and it also addresses the long-term physical, psychological, and psychosocial impacts cancer has on patients throughout their lifetime, and their families, support systems, and care teams." We are so proud of this document, and it will serve as a convincing argument for getting pediatric cancer written into the Wisconsin Cancer Plan, 2030-2040. The reason why this is such a big deal is that very few states even recognize childhood cancer in these plans, and not every state has a specific action plan devoted to childhood cancer. Thus, this certainly puts Wisconsin on the map for recognizing and being a champion for childhood cancer, and that makes me incredibly proud of my home state.

<u>American Cancer Society</u>:

The American Cancer Society (ACS) is the "leading cancer-fighting organization with a vision to end cancer as we know it, for everyone." I have been working with this organization since 2017 in various capacities. In September 2018, during Childhood Cancer Awareness Month, I had the incredible opportunity to step onto the field at a Milwaukee Brewers game with the American Cancer Society. I met some of the players, accepted a check for childhood cancer research from one of the coaches, and listened as my story was shared over the loudspeakers throughout Miller Park. As a Brewers fan, it was a thrilling experience!

Furthermore, I co-chaired and organized the Fashion for a Cure fundraiser in September 2019, which was a fashion show for childhood cancer patients, survivors, siblings, and friends. This was the first childhood cancer fundraiser for ACS in the La Crosse area. In addition, I was an active member of the Chaseburg Sole Burner committee, which was one of this state's most lucrative fundraisers for ACS, from 2018-2021. I was also honored to serve on the State Leadership Board in Wisconsin from 2019-2021. Finally, I currently serve as one of ACS' Voices of Hope, which are "empowered cancer survivors and caregivers who speak about their cancer journey to inspire others to support the mission of the American Cancer Society. Voices of Hope are speakers who offer inspiration to cancer survivors, caregivers, family, and friends, while encouraging involvement with the American Cancer Society."

<u>Gold Together for Childhood Cancer</u>:

Gold Together for Childhood Cancer is the American Cancer Society's childhood cancer initiative, with all funds directly supporting childhood cancer research, advocacy, and patient care. It was founded by childhood brain cancer survivor Cole Eicher and his mother, Laura. Cole started by creating a Gold Together team at his Relay For Life event in

St. Petersburg, Florida, with a vision of expanding to every Relay event nationwide. While still in high school, he founded Gold Together, which became an official ACS initiative in 2018. The movement aims to raise funds and awareness, support patients and survivors, and connect families to lifelong ACS resources. Cole and Laura, now dear friends and colleagues, are incredibly positive and resilient. They are true symbols of *hope over despair.*

While I have volunteered in many roles with the American Cancer Society, my passion for childhood cancer led me to get more involved with Gold Together. I chaired Wisconsin's first Gold Together team in 2022 and soon after, joined the inaugural Gold Together Advisory Council, where I continue to serve. The Council promotes childhood cancer awareness through advocacy, social media, campaigns, and fundraising. As one of the advocacy co-leads, I mentor high school students, teaching them the foundations of advocacy and helping them build the confidence to speak effectively with legislators and others. It's truly rewarding to watch these young people grow into empowered advocates.

In addition to mentoring students on advocacy, we also guide them in their fundraising efforts. I've learned so much from their creativity. It's inspiring to see the bold, innovative ways some of them raise money. Others, like me, may be more reserved, yet they still find clever and effective strategies to support Gold Together. Beyond advocacy, I contribute ideas, resources, and content to the Advisory Council and have helped create and edit materials for various campaigns. Though we typically collaborate virtually from across the country, we've had the opportunity to connect in person at CureFest for Childhood Cancer in Washington, D.C., where I've participated from 2022 to 2024. It was a meaningful chance to work together face-to-face and hold impactful workshops.

CureFest for Childhood Cancer:

CureFest for Childhood Cancer is a national gathering held in Washington, D.C., bringing together childhood cancer patients, survivors, families, caregivers, advocates, professionals, and supporters. The event features workshops tailored to survivors, siblings, bereaved parents, and current fighters, along with opportunities to connect, collaborate, and build community. A Tribute Wall honors both those lost to childhood cancer and those who have survived, while nonprofit organizations participate in a Meet-and-Greet tabling event. An advocacy rally to the U.S. Capitol highlights the need for greater awareness, education, and research funding. One evening features a variety show, with speeches and performances by survivors, patients, advocates, sponsors, and medical professionals.

CureFest not only raises awareness and unites the childhood cancer community, but it also powerfully honors those we have lost. The Candlelight Vigil follows the variety show, during which the names of children who have died are read aloud and echoed by the audience. The Washington Monument Shoe Memorial includes 1,800 pairs of shoes, each representing a child lost to cancer annually in the U.S., placed at the base of the monument. While deeply emotional, these memorials are essential, ensuring these children are remembered and their stories are never forgotten.

Attending my first CureFest was incredible for many reasons. I was continually reminded that some of the best people I know are part of the childhood cancer community, people I now consider my friends, my community, and truly "my people." There's a deep sense of comfort and understanding when I'm with them. I do not have to explain certain parts of myself like I often do outside this space. That kind of unspoken connection is incredibly refreshing.

The camaraderie among childhood cancer patients, survivors, and advocates is powerful and lasting. The friendships formed at CureFest extend far beyond the event itself. They are lifelong bonds. Witnessing the support and connections that CureFest fosters was inspiring, and I often think about how much I would have benefited from something like it as a teenager. Just meeting one fellow survivor back then would have meant the world to me.

Except for the time that I have worked with childhood cancer nonprofits, I did not know anything was available to me because, as an older survivor, it either had not existed, or by the time something was available, I had already aged out of the programs. I did not have any nonprofits, the Internet did not exist as we know it, and I did not meet another person who had neuroblastoma until 2016. This is a terrifying, lonely, emotional, isolating road that few understand, and it can lead to depression, anxiety, and other mental health issues. This is why I am so passionate about survivorship and providing important tools to help survivors have better lives and a better quality of life. I want to improve the lives of survivors to make sure that their experiences are just a bit better than what was available to me and from what I experienced. CureFest certainly fulfills these goals for many, and I cannot express how thankful I am for the opportunity to attend as a nonprofit professional, but more importantly, as a neuroblastoma survivor.

Yet, it is important to further discuss the voice of childhood cancer survivors, who have often had to wait their turn and sometimes fight for a voice in this community. As I have worked with numerous nonprofit organizations, broadened my network of medical professionals and survivors, compared different medical institutions that specialize in neuroblastoma and other pediatric cancers, and compared institutions that have childhood cancer survivorship clinics, I have seen that the voice of the childhood cancer survivor has largely been missing from many places, especially a survivor like me, who was diagnosed in 1980. I have also seen that at times and in certain situations, it can be a long and difficult process to get the survivorship voice out there and to have others listen to and understand that voice. It is exciting to see how that has changed since I began my childhood cancer nonprofit work in 2016, and until the present day. As more children are surviving cancer, it will be important to continue with these changes so that we can support survivors and the challenges that they face throughout their lives.

Coalition Against Childhood Cancer:

One of my deepest goals in life is to fight childhood cancer, especially neuroblastoma, and to help survivors and their families feel less isolated. Growing up, I struggled with that loneliness, and I want others to know what to expect as they navigate a lifetime of survivorship. As the Survivorship Lead for the Coalition Against Childhood Cancer (CAC2), I have the opportunity to address these issues through meaningful programs.

CAC2 is a membership-based organization that includes individuals, nonprofits, corporations, and students from 41 states and nine countries. Members support a wide range of childhood cancer causes across five pillars: Advocacy, Awareness, Research and Treatment, Family Support, and Survivorship. The organization fosters collaboration and provides learning opportunities for members to grow together. In my role as Survivorship Lead, I lead two key initiatives: the CAC2 Survivorship Toolkit and Better Together: Survivorship Connection.

The CAC2 Survivorship Toolkit is a centralized library of educational resources designed for survivors and their families, covering the broad range of challenges they may encounter. My co-creator and I recognized a gap in comprehensive survivorship support. While some toolkits exist, they often focus on only a few topics. Our goal was to build something more comprehensive and extensive. The original Toolkit included over

500 resources, and we will be adding nearly 200 more resources in December 2025 in Version 2.0. Rather than duplicating existing efforts, we spotlight high-quality resources from trusted organizations, while also developing new content to fill critical gaps where little or no information exists.

Survivors and their families often have several issues to contend with post-treatment, including physical and psychosocial late effects, financial hardships, complicated family dynamics, and many more. The CAC2 Survivorship Toolkit draws together expertise from professionals and experienced advocates to create a dependable library of resources and provide "Guidance Along the Survivorship Journey" for survivors and their families. When the CAC2 Survivorship Toolkit working group originally convened, we created a list of challenges and difficulties faced by childhood cancer survivors and their families. That original list mushroomed into an 8-page, single-spaced document that seemed pretty daunting to address. However, that entire list fit neatly into what became the six different categories of the Toolkit: Educational Guidance and Planning; Insurance and Financial Health; Physical Health and Late Effects; Psychosocial and Emotional Health; Transitioning to Adulthood; and Wellness and Healthy Behaviors.

The other survivorship program at CAC2 came about after meeting Carolyn, a member of my "Inner Circle" and fellow childhood cancer survivor, in 2019 at the CAC2 Annual Summit in Columbus, Ohio. At the time, I was nearly a 40-year childhood cancer survivor, and Carolyn was a 26-year survivor, and we met, connected, and formed a special friendship. We realized that even though we did not have the same form of childhood cancer and even though we were diagnosed at two very different ages in our lives, we had a lot in common, and we understood and were first able to bond over being long-term childhood cancer survivors.

It was wonderful to talk and connect with Carolyn because, for most of my life, I never knew another long-term childhood cancer survivor. Also, as previously discussed, survivorship resources have been virtually non-existent for the majority of our lives. Essentially, both Carolyn and I grew up as survivors fending for ourselves. We both felt loneliness, frustration, and isolation throughout our lives as survivors because we did not have access to supportive resources. As a result, the two of us, along with a few others from CAC2, created Better Together: Survivorship Connection, based on the premise that we are "better together." We wanted to ensure that this community had access to organizations that offer current programs, assistance, and support services for the various challenges faced by survivors, their families, and those who work with this population. We both felt strongly that we did not want current survivors to go through what we did and, as a result, experience loneliness, isolation, and a lack of resources.

Better Together provides a database or directory of childhood and adolescent/young adult (AYA) cancer nonprofit organizations that offer programs, services, and assistance for these survivors, their families, and the professionals that come into contact with survivors. By listing all these resources together in a searchable database, Better Together can help families reduce the time spent looking for help when they need it. Furthermore, searches can be personalized, and users can search by specifying the diagnosis, geographic location, and/or type of assistance required. The categories for Better Together that address the various challenges faced by survivors and their families include: Advocacy and Awareness, Disability, Educational Resources, Emotional Support, Employment, Financial and Legal, Flights, Health and Wellness, Home-Living Expenses, In-Person Support, Information, Medical Bills/Insurance, Medical Care/Late Effects, Online Support, Peer Support, Psychosocial Support, Transitions in Care, Travel Expenses, and Wishes and Experiences.

To support our Better Together program, we created the Childhood Cancer Hub, a searchable online database that includes both Better Together and the Hope Portal. While Better Together focuses on resources for childhood cancer survivors, the Hope Portal is designed for those currently in treatment, as well as bereaved families. Our goal with the Hub is simple: no matter where someone is in their childhood cancer journey, they are not alone and should be able to find the support they need through these directories. There is truly something for everyone.

Beyond leading the Survivorship group, I served two three-year terms (2019–2025) on the CAC2 Board of Directors, including five years as Board Secretary and a member of the Executive Committee. This role allowed me to collaborate with and learn from an incredible network of people, both virtually and in person, through meetings, committee work, retreats, and annual summits. Many of these colleagues have become lifelong friends.

I have also been humbled to receive recognition for my work. In 2022, I was awarded the Bob Piniewski Volunteer of the Year award for my contributions to the Board and the Survivorship Interest Group. In 2024, our Survivorship Toolkit Working Group received the same award for launching the Toolkit. Furthermore, among the most memorable experiences during my Board service was being invited, twice, to the White House with fellow childhood cancer advocates. It was a profound honor to have my voice included in such an important space.

I continue to serve as the Survivorship Lead for CAC2, which remains close to my heart. The CAC2 Survivorship Toolkit and Better Together programs feel like my children. I want to ensure they are fully supported and someone is ready to take them over before I step down. Both programs required immense dedication and complement each other, so it would be heartbreaking if either folded due to a lack of leadership. In

2025, I traveled extensively to promote these programs at multiple conferences across the survivorship community. I have also attended and exhibited at events for pediatric hematology/oncology nurses (APHON), social workers (APOSW), child life specialists (ACLP), and palliative care professionals (AAHPC), all of which are key audiences who can get these survivorship programs into the hands of survivors, their families, and the professionals helping this population. I spoke about the Toolkit at the APOSW conference, and I also presented both the Toolkit and the Childhood Cancer Hub at the 2025 CAC2 Annual Summit in Washington, D.C. These efforts are part of a broader marketing push that includes webinars, podcasts, blogs, emails, and additional events.

Not only has working with nonprofit organizations given me a sense of purpose in life, but I have truly met my community and finally feel like I belong. There is so much I usually have to explain about my health, but those in the childhood cancer community already understand. Unlike the general public, they do not need the same explanations. Furthermore, those working in the childhood and AYA cancer communities are some of the best people that I have ever met. I have made lasting, lifelong friendships with fellow volunteers and survivors throughout the nonprofit organizations that I have had the pleasure and honor to be a part of and to serve.

Conclusion

We've all faced difficult experiences, and we all have the choice to let them break us down or permit them to teach us powerful lessons. I believe my own hardships stemming from my neuroblastoma diagnosis and the ongoing late effects I live with have given me a deeper sense of wisdom and purpose. I feel truly fortunate to be involved with several nonprofits where I can support childhood cancer patients, survivors, and their families. Still, this work can be emotionally heavy, as I am constantly confronted with stories and images of brave children who are battling cancer, have passed away, or are survivors still suffering from the long-term effects of treatment.

Researchers are not only seeking cures but also striving to create therapies with fewer and less severe late effects, so survivors can live healthier, more fulfilling lives. I deal with many late effects, largely due to the timing of my diagnosis, the treatments I received, and the nature of my tumor. While some advances like immunotherapy have emerged since then, the development of chemotherapy drugs specifically for childhood cancers remains limited. As I mentioned earlier, nearly all of the chemo drugs I received are still in use today, except for one. This stagnation is driven in part by the lack of financial incentive, as childhood cancers are far less common than adult cancers. But what is often overlooked is the immense number of life years saved when a child survives cancer. And that is something both the industry and government must start prioritizing.

Since I have thrown myself into fighting childhood cancer and using my story as a neuroblastoma survivor to try and bring some hope and help to people, I have had the opportunity to meet some amazing people from all over the world, and do very meaningful, important work. I almost feel selfish because I feel so enriched and fulfilled, and I get so much out of the work that I do. My philosophy and mentality behind my book is finding hope and positivity in any situation, no matter how terrible or difficult it may be. Though cancer and the late effects are truly horrible and devastating, I have found my purpose and passion, and I have had the honor and pleasure of working with many fighting against childhood cancer in a variety of ways. I am hopeful that we can make a difference in the survival of all childhood cancers in the future.

You can decide to focus on hope, optimism, and positivity, even when it feels next to impossible. Even the smallest "silver lining" can be identified and spark some hope. This mentality and the mantra of trying to purposefully live with "hope, optimism, and positivity" have been important for me because it has helped me to avoid becoming too sad and depressed at certain points in my life. Furthermore, you are not expected to be a happy, positive, optimistic person who is full of hope at all times. It is just not practical. Yet, you can start implementing pieces of it here and there, and explore different options and ways of doing things that are perfect for YOU.

I have been asked a few times about the advice that I would give to a family whose child had just been diagnosed with cancer. As I have pondered over this question, I have eventually realized that my advice to those newly diagnosed with cancer would be the same advice that I would offer to a childhood cancer survivor, and at every stage in between. No matter how difficult and dark life can get, especially throughout the diagnoses, treatment, and survivorship of childhood cancer, always try to look for hope, for something positive, and even the smallest sliver of a silver lining in even the darkest of situations. I believe that having hope, even the smallest amount, can help get you through the many challenges of life, from the more mundane, routine experiences to the ultimate stressor of childhood cancer and all of the feelings that accompany this diagnosis. This can be accomplished through not only finding hope, but also finding positivity and optimism in any situation, as well as having faith, humor, kindness, love and support, an outlet, and practicing gratitude, kindness, and giving back.

Overall, I was diagnosed with neuroblastoma at a time when there was little hope for survival, but I feel like I survived for a reason. I want to use my story and provide hope, support, and encouragement to those touched by cancer. Furthermore, I also hope that my work with these and other nonprofit organizations makes a difference in the awareness, support, advocacy, and research for all types of cancer. I hope that it also inspires you to become involved in some way, such as volunteering with or donating to a childhood cancer nonprofit organization. Finally, whether you are facing a trivial issue or childhood cancer has just been introduced to your family, it is important to try to change your perspective. By allowing yourself the grace to live a more positive, optimistic life, you can strive to achieve *Hope Over Despair*.

About the Author

Mariah Forster Olson is an author and passionate childhood cancer advocate dedicated to making a difference in the lives of survivors. Drawing from personal experience and deep compassion, she actively supports children and families affected by pediatric cancer and continues to volunteer with various nonprofit organizations. Through lobbying, writing, and community engagement, she works to bring hope, awareness, and meaningful change.

Mariah can be reached at:
www.HopeOverDespair.com.

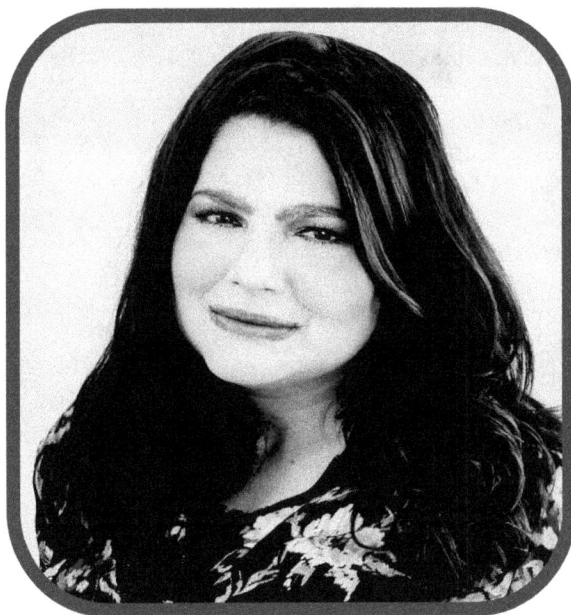

References

ACS Gold Together for Childhood Cancer
Alberta Health Services
All About Jesus Christ
American Academy of Ophthalmology
American Cancer Society
American Heart Association
American Kennel Club
Ask Difference
Asthma and Allergy Foundation of America
Baylor College of Medicine
Cancer Research UK
CatTime
Cedars-Sinai
Centers for Disease Control & Prevention
Children's Oncology Group
Cleveland Clinic
Coalition Against Childhood Cancer
Connecticut Counseling Centers
CureSearch
Dana-Farber Boston Children's Hospital
Dwight D. Eisenhower Presidential Library
Foundation for Medical Education and Research
Fresenius Kidney Care
Ganz, Patricia, "Survivorship: Adult Cancer Survivors"
Help Guide
Icahn School of Medicine at Mount Sinai
Johns Hopkins Medicine
Journal of Clinical Oncology
Journal of Pediatric Oncology Nursing
Kentucky Counseling Center
Mayo Foundation for Medical Education and Research
Medical News Today
MediCopy
Memorial MRI & Diagnostics Imaging Center
Merriam-Webster Dictionary
Micheli, Jason
MyRedeemer

National Cancer Institute
National Institute of Health
National Institute of Mental Health
National Institutes of Diabetes and Digestive and Kidney Diseases
National Kidney Foundation
National Library of Medicine
National Organization for Rare Disorders
Neuroblastoma Neuromodulation
News Medical Life Sciences
OncoLife
Organon Company
Panoramic Health
Pediatric Blood Cancer
Pets Radar
Rasmussen University
Rheumatic Disease Clinics of North America
Ronald McDonald House Charities
Siamese Rescue Group
Sleep Foundation
SpineUniverse
St. Jude Children's Research Hospital
Stop the Thyroid Madness
Texas Children's Cancer Center
The Holy Bible
U.S. National Library of Medicine
U.S. News & World Report
Urology Care Foundation
Verywell Health
Washington Post
WebMD
Wikipedia
Yale Medicine

www.ingramcontent.com/pod-product-compliance
Lightning Source LLC
Chambersburg PA
CBHW062047270326
41931CB00013B/2979